Mamma Gram is a forty-eight year old mathematics teacher. Having experienced a lengthy, stressful time at school, she is unexpectedly diagnosed with breast cancer and suddenly her life is turned upside-down. This is an accurate and factual account of eighteen months of her life as she coped with her diagnosis and treatment, the impact it had on her family and friends and life afterwards. She has written her book with the intention of helping other women faced with a potential life-threatening disease come through the ordeal. All events are true but the names of the people involved have been changed.

The book is written in the form of a diary with lighter hearted moments, illustrations and quotations from various sources. It does not profess to be a medical dictionary but is an autobiography written with hindsight, insight and foresight.

Keeping Abreast Of Cancer

The Not-so Secret Diary

Of Mamma Gram

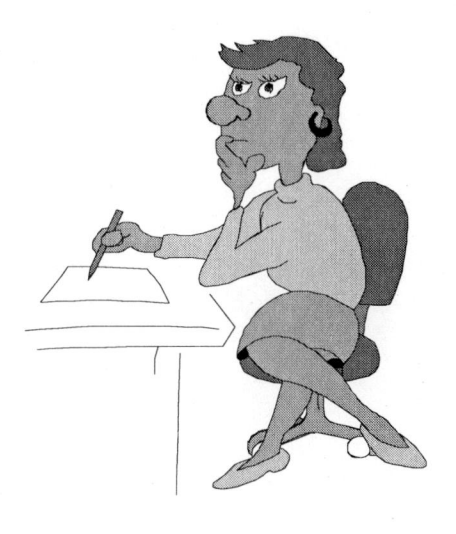

(size 36B → 32A)

Copyright © Jacky Ford 2006
All rights reserved

Contents

Dedication

"To know the road ahead, ask those coming back."
Introduction

"A Prayer For The Stressed"
May – August 2003

"Life's challenges are not supposed to paralyse us; they are supposed to help us discover who we are."
September 2003

"He who has health, has hope; and he who has hope, has everything."
October 2003

"You can only go halfway into the darkest forest; then you are coming out the other side."
November 2003

"Only those who risk going too far can possibly know how far they can go."
December 2003

"In golf as in life it is the follow through that makes the difference."
January 2004

"There are many paths to the top of the mountain but the view is always the same."
February 2004

"As we live, so we learn."
March 2004

"There are no short cuts to any place worth going."
April – June 2004

"A smile will gain you ten more years of life."
July – September 2004

"Today is the tomorrow you worried about yesterday."
October – December 2004

"May your troubles be as few and as far apart as my Grandmother's teeth."
Life Afterwards – January 2005

"It is not about what if, it is about what is."
John's Memories

"Yesterday is history. Tomorrow is a mystery. Today is a gift. That's why it's called the present."
Epilogue

Dedication

This book is dedicated to the Three Musketeers – my husband, my GP and my "adopted big brother" – because, as a quartet, it was all for one and one for all; and to Janet (1947 – 2004) who bravely fought the battles but eventually lost the war.

To you, the reader, I offer the words of an Irish Proverb: "May you have the hindsight to know where you've been, the foresight to know where you're going and the insight to know when you're going too far."

I would like to thank my family, friends and colleagues for their unfailing support during the last two and a bit years even though they all took great delight in having a legitimate excuse for "bullying" me. I must also express my heartfelt gratitude to all the medical staff whose dedication and professionalism were both beyond measure. In particular I must pay tribute to my GP whose understanding and extremely prompt action enabled me to undergo surgery and receive treatment at the earliest opportunity.

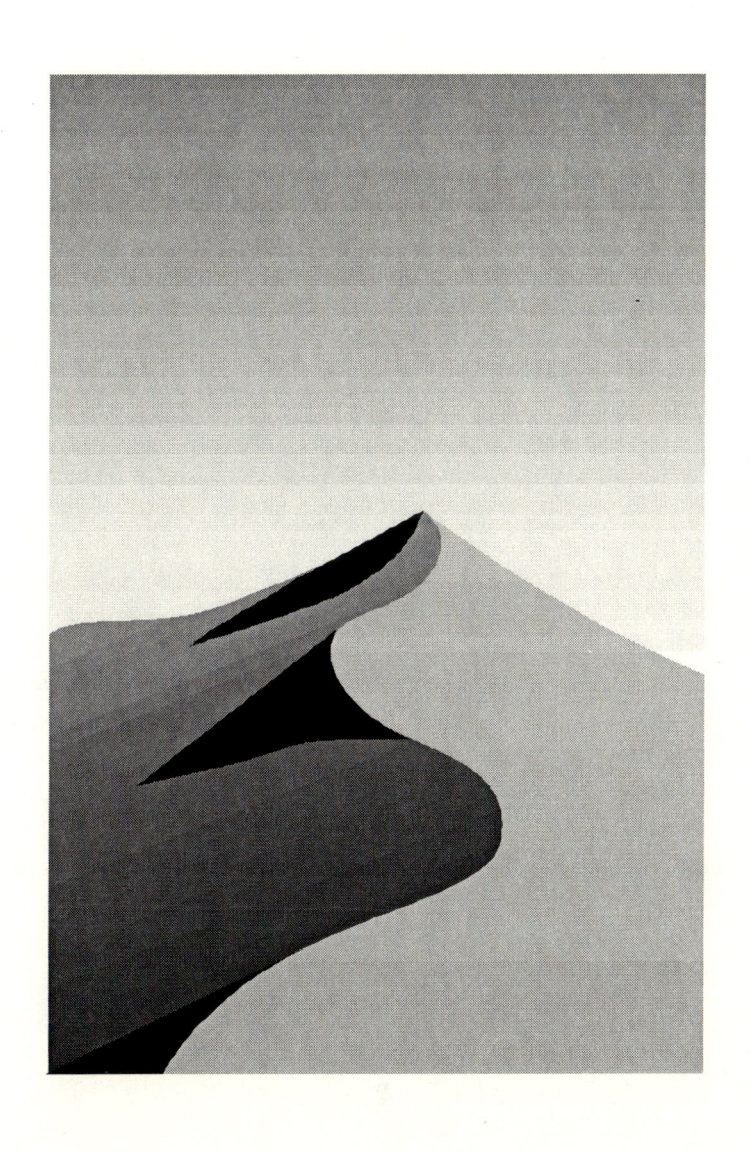

"To know the road ahead, ask those coming back."

Introduction

My name is Mamma Gram (my parents have a strange sense of humour) and I am forty-eight years young. The year 2003 was not particularly kind and, to be perfectly honest, part of me could not wait to see the end of it. The "Outlaw" (a.k.a. the mother-in-law) had undergone heart surgery in March; for the second time in her life, my mother lost a brother to cancer in the summer. In September my husband's cousin also died from cancer despite putting up a brave and remarkable fight against the disease for a number of years.

I live in the southwest of England and am an Assistant Head teacher in a secondary school for students aged eleven to sixteen (you know – the really awkward age). My specialist subject is mathematics (this revelation usually kills a conversation as people say they were never any good at the subject when they were at school!). During the last five years the mathematics department has experienced various staffing problems and, on four separate occasions, I had to take on the extra responsibility of Acting Head of Department. Working an average of fifteen hours a day, usually six days a week just to keep on top of everything, my body, seemingly without consulting my brain, decided enough was enough. My usual "safety valve" of having a migraine attack once or twice a year had ceased as I told myself I did not have time to be knocked out for a day or two. By the middle of May friends at school took it upon themselves to contact a couple of governors to express concern over my state of health. Being a fiercely independent person (my mum would say pig-headed) I did not appreciate what I considered to be their interference. However, hindsight is a wonderful vehicle that provides us with 20/20 vision and I now know I owe them a great deal.

In just over twenty-six years of teaching I had been absent through illness for a total of roughly three working weeks. I was the sort of person who saw their dentist more than their doctor and that was only twice a year for a check-up. I have a very real phobia regarding surgeries and hospitals, to the extent that my parasympathetic nervous system takes over control – ice cold hands, followed by sweaty palms, stomach feels as though it belongs to someone else, frequent need to visit the bathroom. So, unless I was feeling almost at death's door, visits to the doctor were strictly rationed! In fact, I prided myself on the length of time between visits. In fairness I must point out that my doctor is absolutely superb and understands it is nothing personal against him – it is simply the result of some very traumatic experiences as a child. Therefore, when I was suddenly diagnosed with breast cancer, I had no idea what to expect at any stage during my illness.

My purpose for writing this book is to share my experiences, thoughts and feelings so please feel free to help yourself to as much or as little as you wish. Although this is my diary do not be afraid to turn the pages or feel you are intruding at all. I was not the first woman to step into the unknown and I won't be the last. Remember that you will react to your diagnosis, treatment and life afterwards in your own unique way. There is no prescriptive code of behaviour other than to try to be honest and true with yourself because **you** are the most important person in all of this.

During the last eighteen months I have learnt much about breast cancer that undoubtedly enabled me to cope with various situations. My one piece of advice to anybody diagnosed with any form of cancer would be to ask questions at each stage as the medical staff were brilliant at explaining procedures, treatments, effects etc. Nothing I asked was ever deemed too trivial and they must have been subjected to the same questions thousands of times.

What follows is a diary of events as they unfolded. I hope that readers will be able to identify with certain entries and take some comfort that others have felt the way you do and you are not alone. Be reassured that there **is** life after cancer – after all, I have been there, done that and bought the T-shirt! Oh yes – and written a book! Not bad for someone used to numbers and sums. Survivor is one of the greatest words in the English language but I hope to have demonstrated that I am doing more than existing in spite of the cancer.

Finally, in the words of Mao Tse-tung, "A journey of a thousand miles starts with a single step."

Wishing you everything you wish yourself.

Mamma Gram
January 2005

PS Confession time. You need to know that I have been a Tottenham Hotspur Football Club supporter since the age of eight and the only TV soap programme I watch is Neighbours, hence the references in italics to the character Stephanie Scully. Sad but somebody has to do these things!

PPS I am not responsible for the three news items dated 10 March, June and 26 September. I found them on the website.

PPPS All the events are true but I decided to change the names to protect the guilty, including myself!

A Prayer For The Stressed

Grant me the serenity to accept the things I cannot change, the courage to change the things I cannot accept and the wisdom to hide the bodies of those I had to kill today because they got on my nerves.

And help me to be careful of the toes I step on today as they may be connected to the feet I may have to kiss tomorrow.

Help me to give 100% at work
12% on Monday
23% on Tuesday
40% on Wednesday
20% on Thursday
And 5% on Friday

And help me to remember
When I'm having a bad day and it seems that people are trying to wind me up, it takes 42 muscles to frown, 28 muscles to smile and only 4 to extend my arm and smack someone in the mouth.

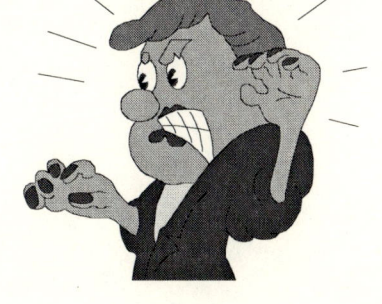

May – August 2003

As it turned out Friday 23 May was one of the most significant days of 2003. A colleague said she needed to talk privately to me about something and asked if we could go to my office. She started by saying she had a confession to make and hoped I would not be cross. As this member of staff is one of the most efficient and conscientious people I have ever worked with, I was totally unprepared for what followed.

The previous evening she had spoken to the Chair of Governors about the pressure of work I was under and the effect it was having on my health. Friends on the staff were worried I would suffer a breakdown if the situation did not improve. She also showed me a copy of the letter she had written to the Head teacher. I said I was not cross, appreciated her concern but needed to make an urgent phone call. After she left the room I rang one of the school's Governors (who is also a vicar) and asked if he would come to school to collect me as my husband was out of the country on business. Within ten minutes he appeared in my office and told me to gather my things together while he cleared me leaving the school site.

Much of the rest of the day, which I spent at the vicarage with the vicar and his wife, is a blur. I was mentally exhausted but, even though I had not been able to sleep for more than three hours a night for many weeks, did not feel physically tired. A close staff friend was "summoned" to the vicarage to be with me and, other than refusing point-blank to be taken to see my doctor (surprise, surprise), I cannot remember anything else that happened. (Several days later I learned that four staff had already shared their concerns about me with the vicar so my early morning phone call to him had not come as a complete bolt out of the blue.)

Somehow I made it through to the end of the summer term – I think I must have been on autopilot much of the time as there are many gaps in my memory. Various people tried to persuade me to consult my doctor but, being a "medical expert", I dug my heels in by saying I was fine and stubbornly refused. After all, who knows my body best? Me of course! Then, one morning near the end of term, I looked in the mirror and was shocked to see the somewhat gaunt face staring back. I felt I was losing my identity and spinning out of control. At that point I decided I had to dig really deep inside me and arrange a visit to the doctor's at the start of the holidays.

Apart from myself, only the "Three Musketeers" know how much that visit cost me in terms of mental anguish. Driving to the surgery the parasympathetic nervous system kicked in as usual. However, I did not have time to report to the receptionist as my doctor spotted me and ushered me into his room. He remarked it must be something serious, as he had not seen me in the surgery for a long time. That actually gave me the opening I needed to explain the pressures I had been working under, lack of appetite, the three hours sleep every night, waking up feeling totally alert, brain always on the go, the inability to switch off or concentrate for any length of time, the music which kept popping into my head. Emotionally I felt extremely drained. He asked me to talk through a typical working day. Well, I was at school by half past seven every morning, usually worked through the lunch break, had meetings after school at least twice a week, left at six o'clock on a good day and then worked during the evening often until after ten o'clock stopping only to eat a meal.

We then pursued leisure time or rather the lack of it. If my husband was playing in a golf competition on a Saturday I either worked at home or went into school. On a Sunday I tried to play golf whenever possible. The next question was how long had I been sustaining this pace – a few weeks? No reply. A few months? I remained silent. More than a year? Yes – nearer four. He took my blood pressure and, amazingly, it was normal. After discussing various options – some feasible, some non-starters as far as I was concerned – I was given a prescription for anti-depressants. I simply hate taking tablets – my throat always seems to close up at the mere thought of having to swallow them. Anyway, the decisions to take the prescription to the chemist's and take the tablets were mine and mine alone. I was assured I had complete control of the situation and reassured I had shown strength of character rather than weakness in facing up to the situation and seeking help.

Apparently the number of doctors, teachers, dentists, lawyers, clergy and other professionals suffering from stress and depression is increasing. Now a statistic I had only myself to blame for not listening to the wisdom of others and acting sooner rather than later. However, at that stage I was unaware of a more serious, potentially life-threatening problem and what lay ahead.

One Saturday morning in early August, sitting in the departure lounge at London Gatwick Airport, I did not feel the usual tinge of excitement before three weeks of sun and golf. At that point I realised I was near the edge of the precipice and made the decision to start taking the tablets.

The holiday provided a much-needed change of routine but I found difficulty concentrating for any length of time and the almost continuous music in my head nearly drove me mad. I have absolutely no idea exactly how many songs I remember the words to but it must be well over two hundred! The tablets made my head feel fuzzy and hands shake slightly – I thought they were supposed to be helping not making matters worse. I suppose I should have realised that it takes time for your body to adjust to medication but, as I have never been patient when faced with illness or injury, I just wanted an instant cure for years of self-inflicted abuse. I needed everything to return to normal so I could resume life at the usual 100mph. I was feeling physically and mentally tired as everything began to catch up with me. Being four thousand miles from home and unable to see my doctor was scary to say the least. Yes – I do realise what I just said – I actually **wanted** to see him to discuss what was happening to me.

The day after we returned home I rang the surgery and was offered an appointment for half an hour later. I hardly had time to think but, upon arrival at the car park, my body felt as though it belonged to someone else and I was on the outside looking in. My doctor remarked that I looked well (a good suntan hides many things) but looks are often deceptive and he was more interested to know how I was feeling inside. The human brain is a remarkable organ – in the space of what appeared to be no more than two seconds I had so many thoughts that I did not know where to start. Although we had been away for three weeks I did not feel properly rested and the tablets were disagreeing with me; I had several tasks to complete before returning to school and could feel the well of pressure beginning to rise again. The tablets were changed and it was suggested I talk to someone sooner rather than later about my workload.

Having been in education before changing vocations, I decided to consult the "Third Musketeer" and ask for his advice on the best way forward. I must admit I was unprepared for his radical suggestions: clear start and finish times at school every day, maximum number of hours worked in a week, having a proper lunch break (I didn't see that one coming!), not working more than five hours at the weekend etc. Whoa – how was I supposed to complete everything? I began to wrestle with my conscience and raise several objections only to be met with the response that, without good health, I would be unable to function, as I so desired. It was also pointed out that I owed it to my family and, more importantly, myself. Think about it and we'll talk again tomorrow!

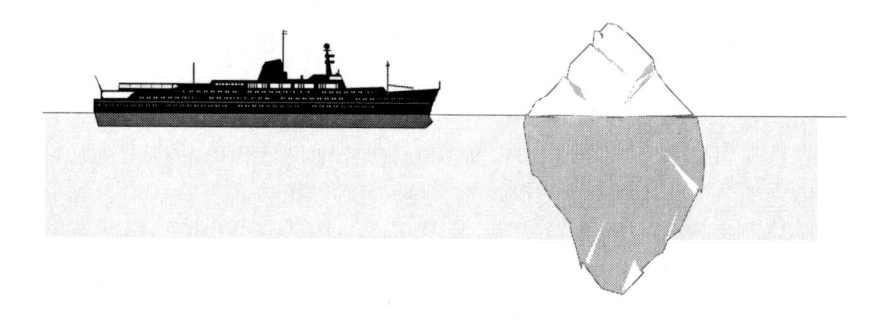

"Life's challenges are not supposed to paralyse us; they are supposed to help us discover who we are."

September

September, the start of the new year in academic terms but, instead of returning with batteries recharged, I was feeling very much out of sorts. Even accepting a dare to wear a particular T-shirt purchased on holiday (which had a witty slogan on it) failed to lift my spirits although it did give certain people a smile. Focusing on tasks for any real length of time was difficult and I seriously began to think my brain was shrinking. Two of the three musketeers appeared to be ganging up on me regarding the number of hours I worked. However, it is hard to change the habits of a lifetime and my professionalism prevented me from easing up.

Wednesday 10 September will be forever etched in my mind. I have a mole on my left breast and that morning it suddenly began itching. My response to skin irritations has always been to scratch them – I have a few small scars where chickenpox and mosquito bites have been "treated" in this way. Needless to say I began scratching the mole and was horrified to find bits of it flaking away. My immediate thought was the years of sunbathing (more often than not without using sun cream) had inevitably caught up with me and I had a melanoma. All day at school I tried to push the negative feelings to the back of my mind but with little success. As soon as I arrived home I "consulted" Jeeves on the Internet about skin and breast cancers and breast self-examination. In the shower that night I plucked up the courage to examine both breasts. The left one appeared to be normal; the mole seemed to have settled down and was no longer causing a problem. However, I thought I could feel a lump on the right breast. Given everything else that had happened in recent months I dismissed it as an overactive imagination.

The following weekend my husband and I played in a local Pro-Am golf competition. Unfortunately, due to fog, our tee time was delayed by two hours. Not enough time to go home and do any work so, as the club did not have Sky television, we watched the Solheim Cup on Ceefax. Sad or what? We rapidly reached the stage where, to relieve the boredom, we were placing bets on how quickly the page would change to update the scores! Perhaps the banality was just what I needed because I played well and won the ladies' prize. Surely, if I had cancer, I would not be physically fit enough to do everything I was doing?

By the middle of the second week of term, I knew the pressure of work was again building up. I was creeping ever closer to the edge and, for once, decided to see my doctor sooner rather than later. I had hardly sat down in his room when he said my eyes were telling him a story of continuing stress and depression and suggested I needed to take time out. I protested that I could not afford to have any time off – the thought of the mountain of work I would return to, having two new staff in the department to look after, deserting students and colleagues etc. was too much to contemplate and would only increase the pressure. In spite of my protestations he gave me a certificate for three weeks off and, as before, told me it was my choice whether I used it or not. His response was that he could only offer advice, he would never force me to do anything against my will but, as one professional to another, asked me to think carefully about the possible repercussions of not having a proper and complete rest with some quality time to myself. I suppose I should have mentioned the mole, the suspicion of a lump and the fact I was losing weight to him but I could not face any more medical problems.

I guess I do not have to tell you that the certificate remains in my possession to this day. My birthday arrived towards the end of the month and coincided with my husband attending his cousin's funeral. (Sadly she had fought and lost a battle with cancer.) I had deliberately organised a parents' consultation day so that I did not have to prepare any lessons! On the other hand I had spent many hours during the holidays coordinating appointments for all the staff, the students and their parents in the school. Friends invited us round for dinner so at least we did not have to cook that evening. One of my presents from my husband was the Jimmy Greaves's autobiography (he used to play football for Tottenham Hotspur and England) and four days later I was lucky enough to meet him at a book-signing event in town.

In some respects the month flew by and, before I knew it, my tablets had almost run out. Thinking that one more month of tablets would be enough I made another appointment with my doctor.

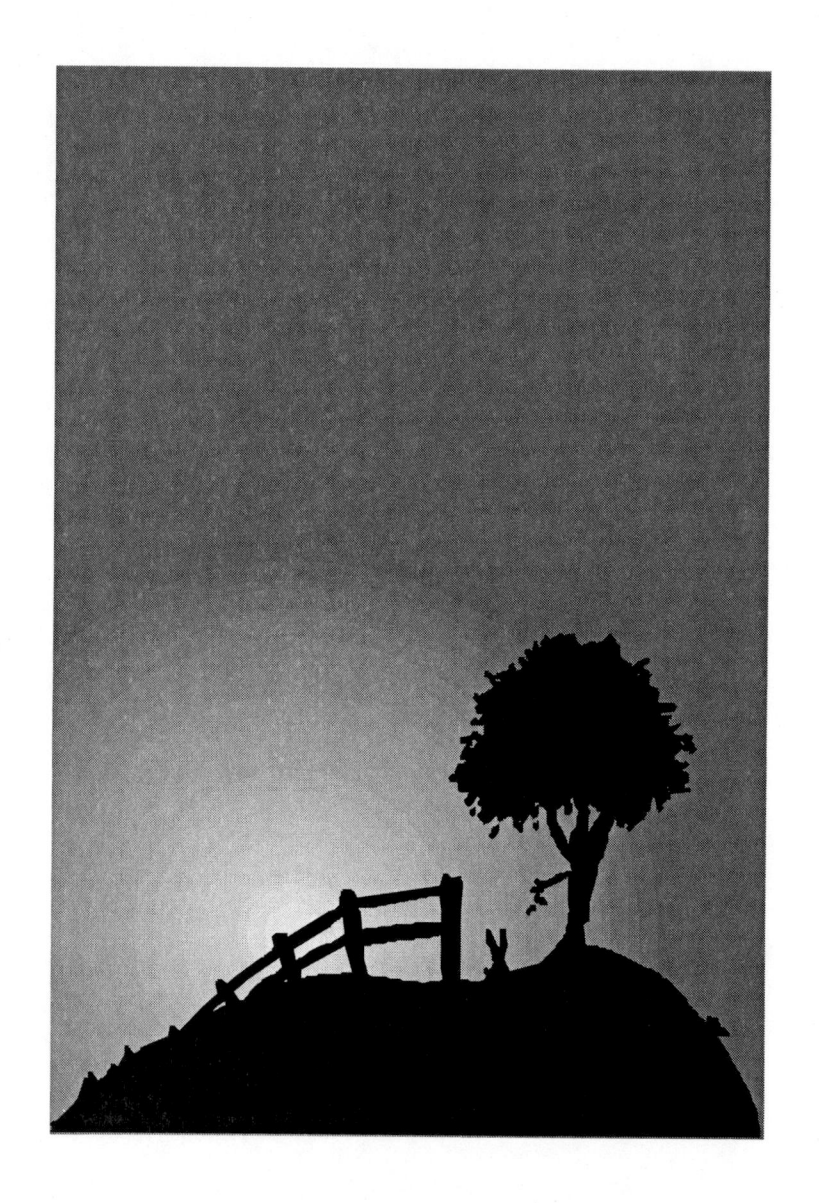

"He who has health, has hope; and he who has hope, has everything."

October

Thursday 2
I saw my doctor today who was not surprised I had been in school every day but he was obviously concerned about me. His professional opinion was I am only just surviving and he wants to know if I lose any more weight. As always he was very understanding, gave me another prescription and again referred to the availability of a certificate. He also asked me if I had thought of harming myself in any way. I was not expecting such a question and it came as a shock but he said it was one he was required to ask. I still could not bring myself to tell him about my ever-growing suspicions.

Friday 3
I had organised a social evening at a local pub for all the staff in my house team. Not feeling in a party mood, it was difficult to keep the mask in place and play mine host.

Monday 6
I examined myself in the shower and I am beginning to feel really scared. I "consulted" Jeeves again and searched two of the breast cancer sites for further information. The more I read the worse I felt as my stomach churned over and over at the prospect I might have the "C" word.

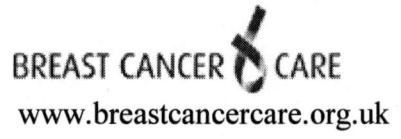

BREAST CANCER CARE
www.breastcancercare.org.uk

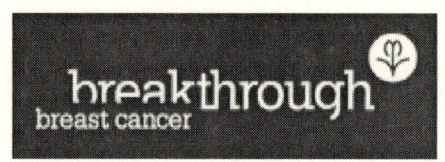

www.breakthrough.org.uk

Tuesday 7
I feel as though I am walking through a fog that shows no signs of lifting. The hours are steadily mounting up again and part of a meeting I attended today felt like the proverbial kick in the teeth. Although I am acutely aware of the possible repercussions, if I am to keep my head above water there is no way I can keep to the proposed work schedule.

Thursday 9
I am now convinced it is not my imagination because the lump definitely feels more pronounced. Next week my husband, John, is out of the country for four days on business. There is no way I can tell him yet of my suspicions as I do not want to worry him. It is only two weeks ago he attended his cousin's funeral. Her illness started with breast cancer but gradually the disease spread to other parts of her body.

Neighbours: Whilst leaning over a car engine Stephanie Scully accidentally discovers a lump on her breast.

Friday 10
The third musketeer, Simon, just back from his holiday, came to see me in my office. He asked me how I was feeling and whether I was adhering to the new routine. I told him about last week's appointment with my doctor, including the question regarding self-harm, before saying I had a more serious problem. Shaking like a leaf I broke down and blurted out what I had found. Typically his calm reply was "So, what are **we** going to do about it? When are you going to see your doctor? Have you told John of your suspicions?" We talked

of my decision not to inform him at this stage and eventually agreed to disagree on my reticence.

Neighbours: Steph decides to consult her GP, Dr Karl Kennedy.

Saturday 11
As John was playing golf I went into school to do some work in my office. However, all I could think about was yesterday's conversation with "my other conscience". For some reason my marriage vows popped in and out of my head – "for better for worse…… in sickness and in health…." Eventually I did some filing and caught up with various letters and emails but it was hard focusing on a task for any length of time.

Sunday 12
I tried to play in a golf competition this afternoon but my head was spinning so much I could not concentrate properly. Whilst in the changing rooms I plucked up courage to ask a trusted friend (who happens to be an ex-nurse and is now a chartered physiotherapist) for a favour. I told her about the lump and asked whether she could give me a simple examination. One look at her face confirmed everything and she told me to see my doctor at the earliest opportunity, tomorrow if at all possible. I collected my bag, put the mask on and found John in the car park.

Monday 13
I rang the surgery and was offered an appointment for twenty minutes later if I could make it. I had just enough time to inform the Office Staff I was going off site and did not require covering. My doctor examined me and said he would refer me for tests as it was not possible for him to determine the exact nature of the lump. He guaranteed the letter would be written and posted that day. He then reassured me by saying that, as our county had an excellent reputation for responding to such

referrals I could expect to hear from the hospital within a fortnight.

As I walked somewhat dazedly back to the car park, the realisation dawned that **a lump had been confirmed** and my life seemed to be flashing before me. I sat alone in the car and tried hard not to panic but to rationalise my thoughts. The television advert about cancer that uses Eva Cassidy's "Fields of Gold" kept popping into my head. The statistics tell us that one person in three will be faced with the disease. What if I am the one chosen from the next group of three people? How would people remember me? What had I achieved in my life? Would anybody miss me? How on earth do I begin to tell my family?

I returned to school and immediately sought out the one person, other than Simon, to whom I had confided my suspicions. As I would need some time off for the tests, he advised me to inform the Head teacher without further delay and offered to accompany me for moral support. Ten minutes later and both men knew as much as I did and were then sworn to secrecy. By the end of the day I was absolutely shattered and in no fit state to attend the Open Evening for Prospective Parents'.

I decided to ring John before supposedly returning to school for the evening. I hated pretending everything was fine and almost cracked up on more than one occasion. Although I was almost out for the count I could not sleep as my mind kept going round in ever decreasing circles. Mentally I went through every scenario possible even to the extent of thinking that I had dreamt the whole thing and would wake up. I tried to convince myself that it was probably just a cyst but in the darkness of the longest night of my life, and without my husband there, I feared the worst.

Tuesday 14
Members of staff have been asking me questions about my non-appearance last night and saying it must be something serious for me to miss such an important school event. I

cannot bring myself to tell them anything until I know for sure. Deceiving so many people is hard but, if this turns out to be a false alarm, I will have saved everybody from worrying unnecessarily.

Wednesday 15
I have endured another long day of pretence to all and sundry. The black bags under the eyes look more like sacks. Thank goodness my mum cannot see me at the moment otherwise I would be going through the third degree interrogation **and** the Spanish Inquisition.

Thursday 16
Once every half-term I chair the School Committee meeting – today was one meeting I could have done without even though the students, as usual, had several constructive ideas to put forward. Simon had been attending these meetings in his capacity as a governor and arrived early to have a chat. I tried to tell him about Monday's appointment as calmly as possible but the strain of the last few weeks overtook me.

    I arrived home after six o'clock to find John in the kitchen making coffee. He jokingly asked me what was today's bombshell from the weekly after-school meeting. The reply was the bombshell had nothing to do with school but me. I explained the events of the last week and my reasons for not telling him. His immediate reaction was to give me a big hug and say he wanted to be involved in everything from now on – no more secrets, promise. We talked about telling the family and decided to keep it to ourselves until we knew one way or the other.

Friday 17
Just as well I confessed everything yesterday because a letter arrived with the name of the hospital plastered all over the envelope. Almost by return of post I was being informed that my initial appointment was scheduled for the following Wednesday. My doctor must have written the referral and

posted it before I left the surgery on Monday! I simply cannot believe how quickly the system has kicked in.

Sunday 19
Part of an email to a close friend: the letter says I could have at least three hours of tests to look forward to. The hands have been blocks of ice all weekend. I just hope I don't have to go into the body scanner – I am not very good in confined spaces. When I had to have MIR scans on my ankle only my legs went in but the noise drove me mad for nearly an hour.

Monday 20
I saw the Head first thing this morning, told him about the impending appointment and reiterated the need for secrecy.

Neighbours: Steph is very distracted at work but won't tell her boss what she has found. Karl books her into hospital for the diagnostic tests.

Wednesday 22
Without doubt, this has been one of the hardest days of my life. My hands went from ice cold to sweaty and back again virtually every ten minutes as my parasympathetic nervous system worked overtime. The appointments were running over an hour late and two women sitting near us had been in hospital together and were comparing their post-operative notes in not very quiet voices. Needless to say I nearly walked out when they got to the double mastectomy part. However, John told me later that they both had good news about their respective check-up, which was a blessing for them.
    A nurse called my name and I followed her into an examination room. She gave me one of those "oh-so-terribly-fashionable-one-size-fits-all-elephants" surgical gowns with the "not-easily-forgotten-flowery-wallpaper-pattern (circa 1900) you used to see in your great-grandmother's front room" to put on. The first "initiative test" was trying to tie it up! The consultant then arrived and felt the lump, said it was a cyst and

he would aspirate it straight away. The news that it was **only a cyst** was an immense relief to say the least. In the blink of an eye life was incredibly good again – I was really cross with myself for panicking unnecessarily and then I suddenly felt tremendously guilty for wasting so many peoples' time. However, the consultant said he wanted me to have a full examination and sent me off for a mammogram and ultrasound scan. I was directed down the corridor to a waiting area where one of the hospital volunteers, herself a former breast cancer patient, offered me a drink and asked if I would like to continue a knitting square somebody had started earlier. Even though my mouth was completely dry I could not face the prospect of hospital coffee. People who know me will not be surprised to learn that I politely declined the knitting, as any form of "girlie handicraft" is not my scene at all! I sat clutching the huge gown around me, in a little world of my own, not daring to make eye contact with anybody, desperately wishing to be somewhere else on the planet.

The mammogram was an experience I will never forget. One look at the machine and I would cheerfully have run a mile but, once positioned between those two pieces of plastic, escape was impossible. Keeping still as instructed was an absolute doddle – I could not have moved even if I had wanted to. The radiographer was very good and kept asking if she could "squeeze" a little more in order to obtain a better picture. I never realised that our "assets" could withstand so much pressure and wish I had taken more notice of the numbers on the counter in front of me! At the end I sighed with relief – I don't know what all the fuss was about – and, feeling quite buoyant now, returned to the waiting room to find three people happily knitting. Well, it takes all sorts to make a world.

About ten minutes later my name was called again. Thinking that I was going for the scan it was a tremendous shock to the system to be unexpectedly ushered into the mammogram room again. The radiographer explained they needed an enlarged image of a particular area on the right breast and the "high" immediately deserted me as I began putting two and two together. Being a mathematics teacher, I concluded the answer was definitely four and not five.

Once the radiographer had finished I put the gown on and was taken straightaway to another room for the ultrasound scan. Ultrasound uses very high frequency sound waves to create a picture of internal tissues. It can be used to find abnormal areas in the tissue or to measure the size of structures in the body. The scan showed I had five cysts in the left breast that they were not concerned about at this stage. However, there was obviously a problem with the right breast because the nurses went into a huddle and talked very quietly. One of them then left the room only to return a short while later with a radiologist, a doctor who understands and interprets scans and x-rays. After introducing herself she asked if she could do another scan. What could I say other than please go ahead? From the position I was laying on the bed I could see the display screen for myself and it did not require a rocket scientist to identify the shadows. In spite of my terror I had known the correct answer was four.

Before performing a fine needle biopsy the doctor aspirated another three cysts that she said were masking the area she wanted to concentrate on and then gave me a local anaesthetic. Whilst waiting for the anaesthetic to take effect she showed me the "gun" and fired it so that I knew what noise to expect and would not jump off the bed in fright. To be honest I was scared stiff by this stage and completely incapable of any movement. The first attempt at the biopsy did not work properly (the "gunshot" was more like a pathetic pop) and so she tried again. Once she had the required sample the needle was removed and a nurse applied pressure on the area for about five minutes. Steristrips were placed over the wound and then covered with a dressing. At last I was able to ditch the gown and, slowly and carefully, put my clothes back on.

I have to return next Wednesday (29th) for the results and be told the next course of action – another biopsy or whatever. I now know what is involved in a biopsy but the "whatever" sounds scary – possibly another step into the unknown. Whilst having the scan I had four staff doing various things to me, including the radiologist, and told them that I needed to visit Marks and Spencer on the way home to buy a new bra. When asked the relevance of that statement I explained I had arrived at the hospital as a 36B and, after everybody's pushing, pulling, prodding and removing bits of me, I had shrunk to a 32A! I felt like a pincushion and dared not drink anything in case I began sprouting like a colander! Somehow it lightened the atmosphere and a nurse asked me if I worked. Yes, I am a secondary school teacher. She raised her eyebrows to the heavens and then nodded knowingly. Her reaction was probably more unnerving than anything else that had happened to this point. I hoped she wasn't thinking I needed brain surgery as well!

We were the last to leave the breast care unit and walked out in silence to the car. John had been sitting in the waiting area, watching people come and go, for a total of three hours; for two of them he was unaware of what had been happening to me. I went through the various tests with him and apologised for not being able to come out to tell him what was going on.

I am not allowed to play golf for a week or so, was told to take it easy for at least twenty-four hours, keep the dressing dry, lift nothing heavy and not bother with any housework! When I relayed all of this to John he laughed about the last instruction as we have someone in to clean the house once a week.

The hospital staff were brilliant and explained what they were going to do at each stage of the assessment. They were so professional and caring in everything they did. By the afternoon I was nearly stir crazy and wanted to go into school for the Parents' Consultation Evening. However, John advised against it. I decided I had to go in the next day to relieve the boredom and feel some semblance of a normal routine as well as an element of being in control of my life again.

Neighbours: Steph has an ultrasound scan and is cross that the technician won't confirm her suspicions.

Thursday 23
By nine o'clock I was dealing with the usual rubbish – some things do not change – Mamma's back in harness. At least it gave me something else to think about. Assuming I had been absent yesterday on a course, a couple of close friends asked me if it had been worthwhile. It was difficult telling them the truth and even harder explaining why I had not said anything before. I was totally unprepared for their reaction to the news. Yes, I had always trusted them but defended myself by saying there had been little point in alarming anybody unnecessarily. At that point I also realised I had to take the lead role and, to all intents and purposes, appear strong for everybody else.

Neighbours: Steph has a biopsy and asks Karl to stay with her, as he is the only person she is allowing to support her.

Friday 24
Thank goodness we broke up today for the half-term holiday as I am completely exhausted. Pretending that everything in my life is fine has been very draining both physically and emotionally.

Neighbours: Steph's worst fears are confirmed.

Saturday 25
Somewhat gingerly I removed the dressing and exposed three bruises. The steristrips still marked the spot of the biopsy incision and, as I peeled them slowly away, I crossed my fingers that I didn't spring a leak.

Sunday 26
My usual Sunday morning phone call home, a ritual since beginning teacher training college, was difficult not least because my mum told me that she had suffered a fall on

Wednesday and ended up in her local casualty department. I almost blurted out that coincidentally I had been in hospital the same day. She asked me several questions about my last ankle injury and we compared bruises, swellings, pain, trying to walk, etc.! I explained some gentle exercises to help with blood circulation and ankle movement and advised her to see a physiotherapist as soon as possible.

Monday 27
I had an appointment with my doctor this afternoon as the tablets ran out yesterday and I am not allowed to run after them. I told him about last Wednesday and thanked him for responding so quickly to my initial consultation. He said he would be thinking about me and asked if I would let him know the results.

Neighbours: Steph is still refusing to tell anybody about her cancer.

Wednesday 29
Last Wednesday was difficult but, in many respects, today was actually worse. Like a yoyo, I went from wanting to know the results to most definitely not wanting to know and back again. Typical woman always changing her mind! Before leaving for the hospital I must have visited the bathroom at least ten times with the last nine being non-productive, as I knew they invariably would be.

As we sat in the crowded reception area I looked around and wondered how many women were there for the screening and how many were, like me, anxiously waiting for their results. My name was called and we were shown into a small office. The consultant surgeon was there and the breast care sister. There was no beating about the bush – the core biopsy had revealed a cancerous, grade two, lobular tumour and the lumpectomy could be scheduled as early as the following week. John took hold of my hand. The consultant explained that a lumpectomy is an operation that removes the tumour and also some lymph nodes under the arm that are subsequently tested to find out if the cancer cells have spread into the lymphatic system. This is a network of vessels which links different parts of the body – if the cancer has reached the lymph nodes, it is more likely to have spread to other parts of the body. The consultant was hopeful I would be able to avoid chemotherapy but could not say for certain at this stage. Having explained the operation procedure he left the room and the sister gave me a few minutes to absorb the news before beginning to outline what would happen next.

Starting today I will have to take Tamoxifen every day for the next **five years** and have radiotherapy to look forward to a couple of months after the operation. Stop right there – tablets for five years – I can't do that! As Tamoxifen reduces the levels of oestrogen in the body and your tumour is oestrogen receptor positive, which means that it depends on the oestrogen hormone for growth, you really have no choice if you want to give yourself the best possible recovery was her reply. She softened the blow by joking that taking these tablets did not prevent me from drinking alcohol if I was partial to a tipple. I asked her how long I would be away from school. I was told that it would be a month to six weeks for the operation and recuperation and then another two months or so for the radiotherapy treatment. My mouth dropped open – I cannot be away for that length of time. Before leaving she gave me a packet of Tamoxifen, a breast care information pack and her card so I could contact her directly should the need arise. Her final words to me were that it was all right to give in to the emotions I would probably feel and there was absolutely no shame in crying. As we walked out I could not help but admire her professionalism and thanked my lucky stars that my job did not entail telling people such life-threatening news.

On the way home we decided to drop into the surgery on the off chance the second musketeer was there. We caught him just as he was leaving for lunch and, being the complete professional he is, he ushered us into his room. Having brought him up to speed with the diagnosis he confessed that he had feared the worst given what I had been through. He wanted to sign me off work there and then but I persuaded him that I needed two days in school after the half-term break to sort out various things. At this point he neatly slipped in that we were talking about six to nine months off work depending on the healing process after the operation and the extent of the follow-up treatment required i.e. whether I needed chemotherapy in addition to the radiotherapy. My life was lurching from bad to worse to off the scale.

I now realise that I am no longer in control of the situation and that is actually the hardest part of all for me to accept. I don't "do ill" very well, hate any kind of fuss and have never been good at taking medical orders so heaven help everybody! This patient will definitely test the patience of any saint, never mind mere mortals.

This evening I went surfing on the Internet to find information on my particular cancer. I discovered that breast tissue is made up of ducts and lobules where milk is made, stored and carried through to the nipple during breastfeeding. Breast cancer starts when a single cell in the breast begins to divide and grow in an abnormal way. So put very simply, invasive lobular breast cancer starts in cells that make up the lobules at the end of the ducts. This type of breast cancer is uncommon and affects about 10 – 15% of all women; it can occur at any age but more commonly in the 45 – 55 year age group. Most invasive lobular cancers are oestrogen receptor positive. Apparently, apart from the cancer cells, the brain can also be affected by a reduction in oestrogen levels, and can be experienced as lack of concentration, forgetfulness and irritability.

- Extreme mood changes, from feeling positive and happy one day to miserable and low the next can happen unexpectedly and for no apparent reason.

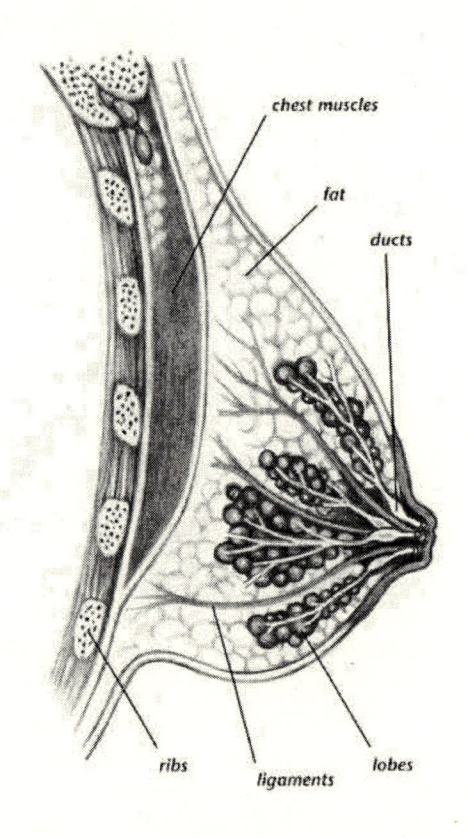

The breast

Thursday 30
I had a long talk with Simon about the events of yesterday. Given my phobia how on earth was I going to cope with a stay in hospital? What if something should go wrong? Suddenly the feeling of my own mortality hit me full force – I felt as though I had been given a death sentence. If anything untoward should happen I wanted him to conduct the funeral

service please, no flowers and donations to go to Cancer Research.

Next problem – how do I tell people at school? I was advised not to do it myself so we sat at my computer and drafted a statement which he would read out on my behalf.

The consultant surgeon rang me at home to confirm the dates for the pre-operative assessment on Monday and next Thursday for the operation. He told me I would be in hospital for two nights. I asked him to aspirate the cysts on the left breast otherwise I feared I would be lopsided! Also I didn't think it was possible to buy a bra with the left cup a different size from the right. Now – there's a thought – perhaps I could design bras for breast cancer survivors?

Neighbours: Steph confides in her best friend, Libby. In order to protect Max, her boyfriend, Steph tells him that their relationship is over.

Friday 31
Hurdle number one – a weekend away visiting my family. First port of call was my sister. While John made sure her children were safely occupied we slipped upstairs to her bedroom. As we sat on the bed I told her that I would be going into hospital next week for an operation as I had breast cancer. Knowing that her sister-in-law also had breast cancer a year or so ago, which had resulted in a mastectomy, I explained everything that had happened and tried to reassure her that my lump had been discovered early. Sarah dissolved into tears with the shock – I guess it is in the job description that big sisters are expected to be around forever! I put my arms round her, swallowed hard several times and promised in a rather shaky voice that I fully intended to be around for each of her three children's weddings, her grandchildren's christenings etc. Her first reaction was to apologise for crying, as she was sure I did not want to cope with people breaking down in front of me. As she usually sees our parents once a week I asked her advice about whether to tell them at this

stage or not. Given their own various health problems she did not feel they were strong enough to deal with news of this magnitude. Now the big question for me is when will it be appropriate? When John spoke to Sarah later on in the afternoon, she appeared to have regained her composure and I had the distinct impression that the two of them were secretly plotting behind my back – not a good sign. As her birthday is in November I almost decided not to leave her card and present behind!

We drove over to my parents and arrived in time to watch the evening episode of Neighbours. Oh boy, talk about the twilight zone – Steph and I have reached the same point today. John and I just looked at each other and dared not say a word.

Neighbours – despite Libby's best efforts she cannot persuade Steph to tell her family or Max.

You know, Steph reminds me of someone!

"You can only go halfway into the darkest forest; then you are coming out the other side."

November

Saturday 1
We went Christmas shopping in Kingston-upon-Thames and the whole population of Surrey seemed to be there. In the Bentall Centre I bumped into an ex-student who had left school several years ago and moved to north London. A ghost from Christmas past – spooky or what! What if this is to be my last Christmas?

Sunday 2
Can now, at last, drop my "Surrey family mask" which has been rather draining. I have spent the weekend looking after Mum and trying to be as normal as possible. I showed her how to do the ankle exercises I had described over the phone and supervised a few sessions.

We drove back home through pouring rain late this morning and I decided to spend the afternoon phoning certain ex-colleagues and friends to tell them myself about the cancer. After the initial shock wore off, I found that people really appreciated being told personally and were unanimous that I had the strength of character – I felt it was their polite way of saying bloody-mindedness – to beat the disease. They all went to great lengths to tell me about family members or friends they knew who had survived cancer and, in particular, breast cancer. One person even mentioned that his grandmother had lived for over thirty years after her diagnosis and that treatment and survival rates had both improved immeasurably since the Dark Ages.

Monday 3

As arranged Simon read out the statement to the staff at the morning briefing. I had specifically asked for cooperation from colleagues rather than sympathy, as I needed to organise certain things and exchange information. However, I could tell individual reactions to the news from the way people looked at me. A wink of the eye here, a crossed finger sign or thumbs up there, friends were respecting my wishes but still able to show their support without crowding my space.

The pre-operative assessment was this afternoon. By the time I reached the hospital my hands were their usual two blocks of ice and my stomach was doing somersaults. The sister asked me questions about finding the lump and the tests I had had. She then told me the purpose of the assessment and said she would measure my height first. I was surprised to learn that I had grown half an inch since 1992 and, no, I was not wearing heels! Next she took my blood pressure, which was normal. Despite my hospital phobia, having an injection or a needle inserted for a blood test has never bothered me, in fact I quite enjoy watching the process. A self-pressurising needle was inserted into my right arm and I filled a phial. The sister removed the phial and replaced it with a second one. The level of blood rose about half way up the little bottle and then stopped. As requested, I started clenching and unclenching my fist to no avail so the needle was removed and the sister remarked that the pathologist would have to make do with what I had given! Apparently I was expected to fill at least three phials! She then indicated the bathroom, produced a small sample pot and I burst out laughing. Absolutely no chance! I had already released enough of my bodily fluids and most definitely was not in a position to pass on any more. Could I bring the sample with me on Thursday morning? With a look of resignation the sister took me down to the x-ray area. Thrillsville – another hospital gown in a paler shade of terracotta to fight with before having a chest x-ray. Man, was the plate cold or what? I now understand the true meaning of "frozen assets."

Neighbours: Steph asks for time off work but is refused so she quits her job. She is refusing to talk to Max in the hope she will drive him away.

Tuesday 4
My last official day in school and the students were asking me why I wasn't teaching their lessons. Having made the decision not to tell them anything until the day after the operation, I replied I was involved in a series of meetings, which was more or less true. It is amazing how easily words trip off the tongue when you are trying to protect people.

Wednesday 5
Day one of my enforced absence and I felt like a fish out of water. Not even a complete day – I was in school for nearly three hours still sorting out various things. I left a farewell message on the staff-room whiteboard and signed it "Love 32A (formerly 36B)" – for people in the know it should hopefully raise a smile.

Trust me, I am a teacher – retail therapy is not all it is cracked up to be. I drove to the large shopping mall outside Bristol and, although I did buy some more Christmas presents, I was looking over my shoulder the whole time expecting to be sprung by a parent from school for truanting! Not possessing any night attire, I also bought a men's pyjama top and shorts set and a lightweight dressing gown. However, I drew the line at purchasing a pair of slippers, footwear I have never worn. This hospital stay has become expensive.

I have done the washing, put it in the tumble dryer, washed my car, sorted out CDs to take with me tomorrow and written some emails. I have played a couple of games of Scrabble on the computer and, due to some of the more obscure words (I'm sure they were in a foreign language) put down by my learned opponent, am suffering from "computer rage". Not that anyone would ever accuse me of being competitive, you understand!

After dinner I thought about packing my bag but then

decided that would bring tomorrow too close for comfort. Instead I played Yahtzee on the computer as I usually manage to beat it!

Thursday 6
Operation Day

Woke up at half past three and, no matter how hard I tried, I could not go back to sleep. The usual trick of working my way around Sainsbury's filling an imaginary trolley with imaginary shopping was unsuccessful so I thought about some of the silly questions of life as any sensible person would. For example, why do scientists call it research when they are looking for something new? If space is a vacuum, who changes the bags and how often? How do you get off a non-stop flight? Eventually I got up, shaved my armpits and legs and then had a shower. Then there was the small matter left over from Monday to attend to. Not being allowed to drink anything meant that producing the required sample was difficult bordering on impossible!

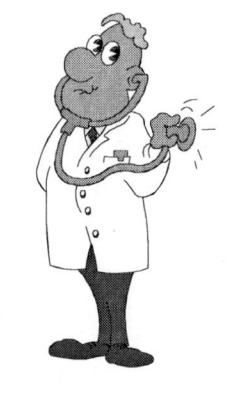

I had to be at the hospital by half past seven, three hours before the operation. The one time I desperately wanted all the traffic lights in town to be red and they were, predictably, green. Some people don't have any luck! After completing the registration formalities with the admissions officer, a nurse came to escort me to my room. A bunch of flowers from my physiotherapist friend and her husband was sitting in a vase on the windowsill.

By eight o'clock I was almost off the planet with fear. The nurse started going through the pre operation procedure which began with me answering the same questions I had been asked on Monday afternoon and concluded with her measuring my legs for the surgical stockings I would have to wear throughout my hospital stay. How embarrassing – that was almost the final straw as far as I was concerned. The green plastic patient identity bracelet was put on my right wrist plus a red one to indicate my allergy to paracetamol. I just needed an amber one to complete the set.

Next to visit me was the anaesthetist. We went through the standard questions and then he asked me if there was anything in particular he should know. Well, the last time I was in hospital to have my wisdom teeth removed, my mum mentioned to the nurse that the hiatus hernia I was born with had never been repaired which was something of a shock to me. (Back in the 1950s most babies did not survive a hernia operation so I had to spend the first two months of my life in hospital waiting for a carpenter to make a special chair for me. For nine months I had to sit upright in a straitjacket, strapped into the chair while the hernia cured itself. I even had to have my nappies changed and sleep sitting up. The straitjacket probably explains a few things!) I pointed out that the hernia had not caused me any problems for over forty years but, straight away, the anaesthetist said he would give me an extra tablet in my pre-med cocktail just in case! In case of what, I wanted to, but dared not, ask him.

The nurse returned and asked if I wore nail varnish. Now, I have never worn make-up in my life – I much prefer the extra ten minutes in bed in the morning – so the thought of nail varnish was quite amusing. She gave me some tape to put round my wedding and signet rings and then produced the made-to-measure size C stockings. The white stockings together with yet another fashionable white theatre gown made me look like a ghost. At least I was allowed to keep my own pants on rather than have to wear those hospital paper ones that are apparently all the rage – not!

I just had time to visit the bathroom to reassure myself that I didn't really need to go, if you follow my drift, before the consultant arrived to mark me up. As well as removing the lump, I asked if he would aspirate the cysts so I had arrows drawn on the right breast and the word cysts written on the left one.

The nurse came in with my cocktail of tablets and the smallest glass of water imaginable with which to try and swallow them. My throat closed up and I have no idea how I actually managed to take them. The clock was ticking relentlessly towards half past ten and the hands and stomach were completely beyond my control. John gave me a card with a message inside "Remember, we're in this together" and a book of Carl Brenders' nature paintings.

A porter arrived to wheel me down to theatre and John held my hand as far as the bottom corridor. He then left to warm his hands on the car heater before driving to Exeter for a site visit; he confessed later that this was really just an excuse to keep active. A nurse accompanied me to theatre as well and asked if I would like her to come into the anaesthetic room with me. I desperately wanted to say yes but was afraid she would think I was a total wimp! The theatre staff took over and started attaching the various wires for monitoring me during the operation. A nurse took my hand to put in the anaesthetic "plug" and remarked that either I had poor circulation or was very frightened. Well, I could definitely guarantee it was nothing to do with the circulation. She then asked if I played any sport. I mentioned golf, heard the anaesthetist say "Slight scratch coming" (why do anaesthetists say that when it is nothing like a scratch?) and then felt the anaesthetic travelling up my right arm. Why haven't they asked me to count backwards from one hundred as they normally do? After all, I am a mathematics teacher. At this point ………..!

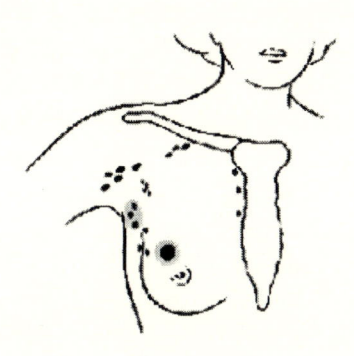

The operation – a wide local excision (lumpectomy) and axillary lymph node sampling (axilla are the glands in the armpit) – lasted over an hour as the clock in the recovery room showed ten past twelve when eventually I came round. I cannot express in words the overwhelming sense of relief from simply looking at a clock but, as I lay there, I said a silent prayer of thanks to my guardian angel. Two hours after the start of the operation I was back in my room and on the phone to Sarah who could not believe I was awake and talking coherently to her. (There's a first time for everything – talking coherently, I mean!) The nurse who came in to check on me was rather surprised as well, as was John who had returned from his business meeting expecting to find me "still out of it". I also rang Simon to let him know his professional services would not be required – well, not yet awhile.

About two o'clock I was brought a pot of tea and asked to order the evening meal. The drink was most welcome as my mouth was drier than the driest place on earth, the Atacama Desert. The tea also caused a problem about half an hour later when I felt the urge to visit the bathroom. Apart from being attached to two wound drains – which remove blood and fluid produced by the cut tissue – I wasn't sure if I was allowed out of bed yet! Now, any person with half a brain cell would probably have called for a nurse but, not wanting to make a fuss, I made a unilateral decision. I swung my legs over the side of the bed and gingerly stood up. No problems – the room didn't spin round so I took four steps forward and came to an unexpected halt as the drains prevented further progress. Not a mistake to make again I thought as I wiped away a tear or six! I lifted the bottles at the other end of the drains and together the "three of us" continued on our little journey. Then the fun started. Why aren't human beings born with three hands? How was I supposed to manage the bottles, my underwear and a flapping surgical gown all at the same time? Why hadn't I refused the tea?

Just before five o'clock I was legitimately out of bed, dressed in shorts and T-shirt, sports socks attempting to cover as much of the hideous surgical stockings as possible, and sitting in a chair watching "Blue Peter" – when did John Noakes and Shep leave the programme? Apart from the two painkillers I was given when I arrived back in my room, I did not have to take any other tablets, which also surprised the staff. No heroics on my part – I genuinely was not in pain so didn't need to take anything.

The night nurse appeared at half past ten to tell me it was now "quiet time" and to mark the level of fluid on each bottle – well, that was the theory. She drew a line about half a centimetre up from the base of one bottle and the other bottle was empty! One of us wasn't at all surprised at the lack of blood and other bits. As I wanted to continue watching the golf from America, she brought me a set of headphones, told me to press the call button when I was ready to sleep and she would return and put the backrest on the bed down.

The hospital staff today were absolutely brilliant – only one minor complaint. I ordered scrambled eggs and smoked salmon for dinner (my tastes are simple) and the eggs looked rather lonely. The clips are due to come out next Thursday and I will be told the results of the biopsies then as well. At this point I gather the surgeon took away a fair amount of tissue and a number of glands.

Friday 7
The first day of the rest of my life

I hardly slept last night because the drains kept getting in the way and I wish the surgeon could come and remove the huge black bags from under my eyes! The nurse came in around 7.30 a.m. to take my blood pressure and check the fluid levels in the bottles – no change from last night. I wasn't surprised at all – bodily fluids are supposed to serve a purpose and my fluids are mine and mine alone. She asked why I hadn't called her to put the bed down.

They (whoever "they" are) say that the most important meal of the day is breakfast but I have managed without eating this meal for most of my life. I don't do mornings, especially early mornings, very well – my stomach doesn't usually start to feel part of my body until lunchtime – but as long as I have my orange juice fix first thing I'm fine. As a small child I had to go into hospital to have my tonsils removed and, on discharge morning, was told by Sister that I wouldn't be allowed to leave unless I ate all my cornflakes. My throat was still very sore from the operation; during my four days in hospital I had seen my parents for just a couple of hours. (Attitudes have changed, thank goodness, and parents can virtually spend as much time as they want with their sick child.) I was absolutely distraught, in floods of tears and will be forever grateful to the nurse who told me not to say anything, took the bowl away and flushed most of the cereal down the toilet returning the bowl just in time. Her kind action meant I left hospital with everyone else but I still feel guilty that I was given an extra sweet for "eating" most of my breakfast. It is strange how a childhood memory could suddenly come to the fore and be so vivid and influential but, not wanting this current stay in hospital to last a second longer than necessary, I forced down some toast with two cups of tea.

After breakfast I decided it was time to have a shower and get dressed. I did not want any visitors seeing me in the pyjama shirt and shorts and it was too hot to wear the dressing gown. I remembered my attachment to the bottles this time and went into the bathroom. Well, the clips and dressings were restricting the movement of my right arm so I changed my mind and had a wash instead. That was difficult enough as I am right-handed and not very good with my left hand. Even worse, I wanted to wash under my right armpit but the drain and dressing were in the way. The left armpit had more sprays of antiperspirant than usual!

About mid-morning the consultant came in to check on me. He looked at the bottles and said the drain to the empty one could be removed after lunch; if the level of the second bottle didn't rise that drain could be removed later in the afternoon. He checked the dressing and offered the option of another night in hospital if I wanted it but felt I was progressing as expected and well enough to go home. No prizes for guessing the choice I made! The consultant said he would see me next Thursday and remove the clips. His parting shot was it would be a sensible idea to keep the stockings on until then just in case of blood clots. Aagh! In the words of John McEnroe "You cannot be serious."

John had escaped from the office and joined me for lunch; surprisingly enough my sandwich slipped down easily. The nurse came to clear my tray away and said she would remove the drain under the armpit. As carefully as possible, she slowly peeled away the dressing only to reveal that a clip instead of a stitch had secured the drain so she would need special scissors. While she was out of the room I asked John to pass me my small mirror so that I could look at the clips. Needless to say the nurse's timing was perfect because she arrived back just as I was admiring the reflection of the neat semicircle of staples in the mirror. It was one of those moments when you had to be there to witness the expression on her face – it was priceless.

I had five visitors during the course of the afternoon one of which was a school colleague. She said that the students had now been told the reason for my absence and were busily making cards.

At twenty past five another nurse came in to announce the removal of the second drain. (Yes – the great escape is fast approaching!) The level of blood and fluid in the bottle had not even reached the bottom of the scale. She peeled off the dressing and commented that the drain was clipped in. As she went to fetch the scissors (which I suppose I could have told her she would need) John began to pack my bag. The clip was removed and, as the drain was released, there was a wonderful slurping noise.

FREEDOM! I was sprung at six o'clock so I only spent thirty-four and a half hours in hospital, not that I was counting of course. I went to pick up the bunch of flowers and a potted plant but was told by the nurse not to lift or carry anything at all. (Earlier in the day I had been told off for lying on the bed with my legs crossed.) The next problem to be dealt with involved keeping the car seat belt away from the tender bits during the drive home!

There is no place like home; I had been away less than two days but it felt like two months. More importantly, I felt I was in charge of the situation again. Little did I know that John had other ideas?

Neighbours: Steph has her lumpectomy. Her brother, Jack, now knows about the cancer.

Saturday 8
Sleep last night was difficult as I kept waking up every time I turned over onto my right arm. It is hard to describe this next bit in words but I have a really strange numb sensation in both my armpit and underneath my upper arm that also feels cold to the touch. I suppose it is an effect of the surgery on the nerves.

The first priority this morning was to have a shower. John insisted on waiting outside the door "just in case" I needed assistance. Not really trusting the waterproof dressings I went through a series of contortions in an effort to keep the soap and shampoo away from them. Drying my hair with the hairdryer was hard work but, as I want my full range of arm movements back as soon as possible if not sooner, I persevered.

Two days of inactivity in a "sauna" (a.k.a. hospital hothouse) and I needed fresh air. I wanted to go into town to do some shopping but my jailer said no. He also refused to pump up my bike tyres. So, just like the vultures in "The Jungle Book" what are we going to do? The jailer suggested doing something that work had prevented for a long time. An old coffee table was set up with my portapuzzle so I could start doing a wolf jigsaw puzzle. As a break from the jigsaw I wrote emails to friends to let them know about my progress so far.

Sunday 9
My usual Sunday morning phone call home and I learnt that my mum had to be taken to hospital on Wednesday night with heart muscle spasms. She had difficulty breathing and said that one side of her face was numb. I think she thought she had suffered a stroke but the tests proved this was not the case. The timing of my illness could not be worse and I feel powerless to do anything constructive to help her at the moment. I hate the idea that I am deceiving my parents by keeping my secret but, deep down, I know they have enough to cope with at present. The jailer eventually took pity and decided to drag me away from the jigsaw. We went for a drive in the car before doing some shopping.

The surgical stockings were driving me wild, made me feel hot and were consigned to the laundry basket. I have been walking around the house and garden on a regular basis and, as the wound drains were virtually empty, I can't see the point of continuing to wear them.

Monday 10
The thousand-piece jigsaw is well under way. I was dropped off at the local newsagent this morning and allowed to walk back on my own. Two friends came round for coffee this morning and I had a stroll in the sunshine after lunch as well. This afternoon I spent over half an hour on the phone to a colleague who is on maternity leave. One of my tutor team, a fellow Spurs supporter, popped in on his way home from school to see how I was progressing. I have done the cover, plus an alternative cover, for my book and resisted the temptation to watch daytime television apart from the lunchtime news and Neighbours.

Gardening has always been a real chore for me and I have a reputation for being able to kill flowers. Courtesy of my various visitors, I have three bunches of flowers (plus instructions – see below) and one pot plant to try and look after. I think most of the flowers are freesias and I have definitely spotted some carnations. As for the rest of them, who knows what they are?

How To Keep Flowers – An Easy Step-By-Step Guide
1. Find a vase.
2. Make sure the end of the vase with the hole is at the top.
3. Put water into the vase. If more help is needed with this ask an expert.
4. Take the plastic wrappings off the flowers.
5. Put the flowers into the hole in the top of the vase. N.B. The long green stick bits go into the water.
6. Check to make sure that the coloured bits (also known as FLOWERS) are at the top.
7. Your flowers are now ready to be looked at and admired. Those people with more experience may even try to smell the flowers.
8. When the coloured bits begin to fall off and lie around on the table, this is a sign that the flowers are beginning to die.
9. When only the green sticks are left the flowers are dead!
10. When the green sticks turn to a brown mush and start to smell really foul, it is time to throw them away. Take care to keep hold of the vase during this operation, as it can be recycled.

WE HOPE YOU HAVE MANY HOURS OF ENJOYMENT FROM YOUR FLOWERS

Also available in this range: Pot Plants – An Idiot's Guide; Cacti – The Plants That Are Difficult To Kill.

Neighbours: Steph's operation is successful but where were her drains and surgical stockings? How come they gave her the results of the biopsy just after she arrived back in her room? Why was she not sitting up and making phone calls two hours after the operation? She is told that she will require both radiotherapy and chemotherapy treatment and the latter could leave her infertile.

Tuesday 11
I was driven to a different newsagent this morning and so had a longer walk home. Simon arrived mid-morning for a caffeine fix and to gently wind me up. Knowing that I would want to run before I could walk, he complimented the jailer on his determined and unrelenting approach to my post-operation care. I promised I would try hard to change the habit of a lifetime and take things easy but was there any chance of him pumping up my bike tyres? It's funny how a single look can say a thousand words.

Not being able to drive the car yet is a real pain and makes me feel more of a prisoner. In the afternoon we went to PC World and bought a new keyboard for the computer. I was unable to attend the Ladies' Annual General Meeting and Presentation of Cups at the golf club. Although I had a trophy to collect we decided it was too soon after the operation to face a large number of people. My apologies were read out and, at the end of the meeting, the Outlaw was asked what was wrong with me.

A close friend and colleague came round after school with some more cards – the parents have now got in on the act. I very much appreciate the messages of support but feel I am being smothered. Phone calls from golfing friends began around six o'clock!

Finished the jigsaw. I cannot remember the last time I had the freedom to spend unlimited hours doing what I wanted to do and not feel guilty that I ought to be doing some work.

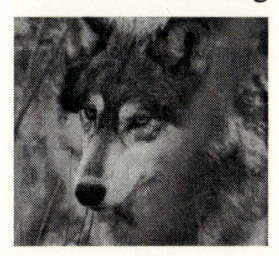

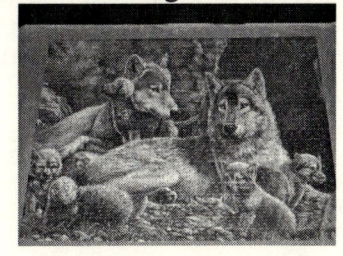

Wednesday 12
The "cavalry" arrived at lunchtime in the form of my physiotherapist and closest friend, Kate. She promised the jailer she would keep me in check before taking me out for a pub lunch. As the sun was shining we had a walk afterwards to burn off the calories from the huge prawn baguette we had shared.

Another milestone reached because today is my niece's seventh birthday. She rang me when she arrived home from school to say thank you for her presents and tell me about her day and forthcoming party. Eventually she paused for breath and then started grilling me about my day at school. I told her I had been busy and had more work to do that night. I am not sure that doing a jigsaw constitutes work but there we go.

Thursday 13
Prognosis Day!

7.20 a.m. I am not a superstitious person, touch wood, but thank goodness it is not Friday the thirteenth! Today is the worst day of all, even worse than when I found the lump, and terrified doesn't begin to cover it because I am completely powerless to change the results. By midday I should know everything. My hands are ice blocks again and my stomach feels as though it belongs to someone else.
9.10 a.m. Yesterday Kate brought me a wasgij – a jigsaw where the picture you see on the box is not the puzzle picture – but my concentration is virtually non-existent and the pieces all look the same. The waiting is tortuous.
11.30 a.m. A nurse took me to a small examination room. She gave me – guess what? – yes, a gown and, while I was changing, went to fetch the consultant. He removed the dressing, looked at the wounds and said the clips could come out. It took the nurse about twenty minutes to remove thirty-three staples – three of them stubbornly refused to leave me and made my eyes water. The nurse asked if I needed a rest

but, as I just wanted everything gone as quickly as possible, I told her to keep going and clenched my fists.

12.00 p.m. The consultant told us that the tumour was just over one centimetre in diameter, which is about the size of your thumbnail, and had been classed as a grade two. The glands showed no further problems and the lymph vessels were clear so the cancer appears to have been confined to one area. I am allowed to drive the car after the weekend and can play nine holes of golf in a fortnight's time. The consultant was unable to tell me about the next phase – the oncologist will see me sometime in the next two weeks to explain about the radiotherapy planning session and treatment and advise me about chemotherapy. We told him that we had already booked a golfing holiday for the February half-term break and did he think I would be fit enough by then. His reply was that the oncologist would be in a better position to answer that particular question. I then asked about the strange sensation I was experiencing in my arm. Apparently it was happening because the nerves running through the armpit were disturbed when reaching the lymph nodes that lay behind them. This had caused trauma to the nerves and it could take up to eighteen months to regain the full feeling although I should be aware that there was a chance I might be left with some permanent damage.

We had to stop at Sainsbury's on the way home to buy a stick deodorant for the right armpit. John rolled his eyes when I told him that I had to buy the same scent as the antiperspirant I usually use! Well, I couldn't have the two armpits smelling differently, could I?

As soon as we arrived home, I dashed up to the bathroom to inspect the scars. The scar on the breast looked like a semi-circle as it followed my natural curve. Both scars were about four inches long, very red and I could see clearly where the clips had all been. I appeared to have a third "scar" – just under the top edge of the areola (the dark area of skin around the nipple) was an indentation and my breast was concave instead of convex. John suggested I should consider having a water balloon implant! No more surgery thanks very much.

By this evening I was feeling very flat for some inexplicable reason. Maybe a delayed reaction had set in because it was difficult to grasp that the events of the last month had been happening to **me**. It felt as though I was on the outside looking in if that makes sense. The fog had closed in somewhat and I couldn't really understand why. After all, the cancer had been removed and the news from the consultant surgeon was probably about as good as it could have been. Metaphorically speaking, I ought to be doing cartwheels like Robbie Keane when he celebrates scoring a goal for Spurs.

Neighbours: Steph is released from hospital and has made the decision not to undergo the chemotherapy.

Friday 14
An ex-colleague from school was in the area visiting her relatives and came round for lunch. She remarked how well I looked just a week after an operation and then gave me a present – a one thousand-piece jigsaw of two collies. "You have time to do these things now!"

Neighbours: Karl counsels Steph to have the chemotherapy.

Monday 17
A friend was due to go into hospital this afternoon and I had promised to keep her company in the morning. **MORE FREEDOM!** I drove the car over to her house although I must admit I felt a bit sore and the seat belt got on my nerves as well as the scars!

Tuesday 18
I had a letter from the oncologist today – my appointment with him is scheduled for this Thursday.

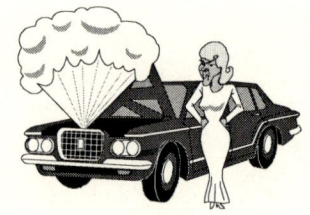

Everything that can be crossed is crossed that I avoid chemotherapy.

Wednesday 19
Another potted plant arrived today courtesy of the ladies at the golf club. The living room is now beginning to look like Kew Gardens in Surrey! I had an appointment with my dentist this afternoon and, as per usual, he asked me about my life down the road at the "learning factory". I explained everything that had happened in the last few weeks and he made notes on my record card. We had a talk about possible follow-up treatment and he asked to be kept informed.

Neighbours: Jack is concerned that Steph is losing the will to live.

Thursday 20
I completed my second jigsaw, sorry wasgij, (where the picture on the box is a clue rather than a picture of the puzzle) and started writing the introduction to my book.

I saw the oncologist (a doctor who specialises in the treatment of cancer using radiotherapy) today. Having had a lumpectomy, the radiotherapy is used to reduce the risk of the cancer coming back in the same breast. I have to go to the Bristol Royal Infirmary next month for a planning session and then five weeks of "being zapped" by x-rays will start in the New Year. He said we should be able to go ahead with our half term holiday as planned. Apparently only two percent of women with similar symptoms to me have benefited from chemotherapy. As the side effects can be very unpleasant and the oncologist doesn't really think I need it, **NO CHEMOTHERAPY** (unless I wanted to insist on having the treatment) which is a huge personal relief. At this rate I should be able to avoid telling my parents altogether.

Although away on holiday for a few days, Simon rang to find out the latest news and offer moral support.

Friday 21
Although nobody else could see my right armpit, I decided I simply had to shave away the unsightly hair. Due to the numbness I could not feel the electric razor on my skin at all (a weird experience) and was particularly careful near the lymph node sampling scar.

Neighbours: Steph tells her family that she has had a lumpectomy.

Sunday 23
The final of the 2003 Rugby Union World Cup: England defeated the defending champions Australia 20-17 (in extra time). I remember watching Bobby Moore, captain of the England Football Team, lift the World Cup in 1966! I choked up then as well.

Monday 24
What a weekend – we are totally exhausted from watching the rugby international, the golf, two football matches and driving to the other side of Exmoor for dinner with friends last night. I am not supposed to be put under undue stress but England and Spurs really did my head in. Thank goodness they both won, even though England left it to the very last kick. John went to work today for a rest!
Finished my third thousand-piece jigsaw today. I have decided to put jigsaws on hold for a short while – you can have too much of a good thing. Instead I am going to start a database on the computer for my stamp collection and First Day Covers. I meant to do this last summer but, for some reason, other issues prevented it.

Tuesday 25
My little sister, Sarah, is "all the fours" today and I was able to ring her and wish her a happy birthday, something I hadn't dared hope would be possible nearly a month ago when I saw her at half-term.

Thursday 27
I was born in Epsom Hospital which is situated not a million miles from Epsom Racecourse, home of The Derby, and I am totally convinced there is a deep, very meaningful connection between my birthplace and intense dislike of horses! I went on many residential trips with students from school and would do just about anything to escape the horse-riding sessions. So, it is incredible to record that I accepted an invitation to go to the races today. Perhaps there are side effects of Tamoxifen doctors are unaware of!

Apart from going to Beanie Babies fairs at Epsom and Ascot racecourses and dry skiing at Sandown Park, I have never had the slightest desire to set foot on a racecourse and watch a race or seven. Along with boxing and wrestling, horse racing really is a sport I can live without. Still, the sun was shining and two very good friends obviously felt the need to further my sporting education.

We had missed the first race, which wasn't a problem as far as I was concerned. I was taken to the saddling enclosure where the horses were parading before the second race and, jokingly, asked to pick the winner. As I know next to nothing about horses I applied my mathematical brain to the task. I thought the grey horse looked well groomed, had the number four on the saddle (my mum's birthday is the fourth of August) and the jockey was wearing pink and blue colours (pink being my niece's favourite colour and Spurs wear blue shorts). Therefore, Beau Torero for me, what do I do next? We walked past the bookies looking for the best odds and I eventually placed a five-pound bet before going into the stands to watch the race. Well, suffice to say that Beau Torero won and I went off to collect my winnings of nearly £19 with someone muttering something about beginner's luck in my ears. I prefer to think it was my sound, oh-so-scientific logic that paid dividends.

Race number three on the card and I was on a roll ... well, one for one. Another grey horse called Daisy Dale caught my eye. OK, number two on the saddle and this was my second race; the jockey was wearing yellow, which is my favourite colour. It seemed reasonably logical to place a bet on this horse and then retire to the stands to watch the race unfold. Until two jumps from the end, Daisy Dale was in the lead but appeared to run out of stamina and finished third. Never mind – now I was down to one for two and time to quit while I was still in profit. I did manage to pick the winner of the next race but the odds were not good enough to place a bet. We watched one more race, race number five, and then decided to beat the mass exodus and leave early.

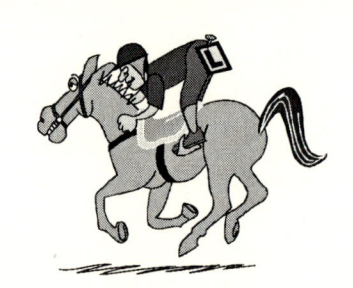

In terms of organisation and completing paperwork the oncologist must be related to my doctor as the Bristol Royal Infirmary has been in touch today. The planning session is scheduled for 22 December and the radiotherapy treatment begins on 6 January. As it doesn't finish until 9 February and we are due to see my parents on Friday 13th I may have my work cut out maintaining my secret.

Neighbours: Max has to take his son to hospital and inadvertently finds out that Steph is having chemotherapy.

Friday 28
Neighbours: Max tells his children about Steph's cancer and treatment.

Saturday 29
We went round to friends for a meal tonight. For the first time since starting the Tamoxifen I had some wine. Cheers!

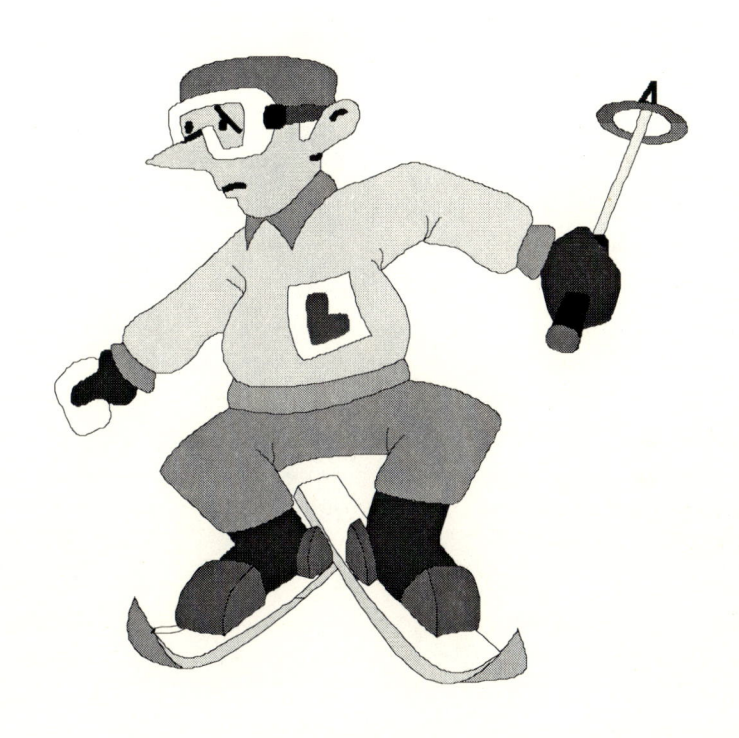

"Only those who risk going too far can possibly know how far they can go."

T S Eliot

December

Tuesday 2
I started my first period since September today. If I hadn't known better I would have been worrying for the past three months that I was pregnant! I suppose the combination of stress, cancer, the operation and Tamoxifen tablets took its toll and perhaps my body is, at last, making a statement about trying to return to normal, whatever that is.

Thursday 4
Today was a real step forward as I played golf for the first time since the Sunday when my worst fears were, in effect, confirmed. I visited the "little room" at least three times before leaving the safety of the changing room. Walking out onto the course I wondered how my body would react. I stood by the first tee and took my driver out of the bag and breathed deeply. Dare I swing the club? What if I split open the scars? Beware the golfer who claims to have a bad back – he/she usually plays the round of a lifetime as the swing is controlled. Now it was a case of beware the golfer recovering from cancer. Almost in slow motion I made a practice swing and then another two or three. So far so good so I teed up a ball and addressed it. I didn't exactly experience a golfer's worst nightmare of suffering the dreaded yips but it seemed ages before I could bring myself to actually hit the little white ball. Relief as the ball sailed down the fairway would be an understatement but suddenly, and inexplicably, I felt very emotional. After seven holes Kate said that was enough for

the first time back on the course. I honestly felt I could have gone further but was not allowed and I almost had to be dragged back to the clubhouse.

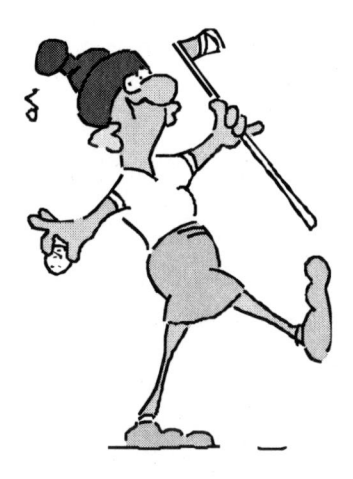

In retrospect I could have hit an easy iron shot on the first tee but, subconsciously, I suppose I was trying to prove something to myself by taking the driver. I cannot sit down and simply let life pass me by.

Neighbours: Steph is losing her hair and this triggers feelings of unattractiveness. She changes to wearing a baggy windcheater instead of her usual close-fitting tops.

Friday 5
Amazingly I did not feel any after-effects from yesterday's golf.

Neighbours: Steph tries to explain to Max that having cancer has turned her world upside-down and she cannot cope with the pressure he is putting on her regarding their relationship.

Sunday 7
My period, which seemed to follow its usual course, finished today. I know that Tamoxifen is an anti-oestrogen i.e. it

blocks the effect of the female hormone oestrogen on breast cancer cells by slowing down or stopping their growth. I have read that it can have side effects including menopausal symptoms such as hot flushes, weight gain, vaginal dryness and mood swings – the heck it does! I am not ready for the change of life yet.

The advice from the hospital was to try to do a little more physical activity each day. I gradually increased the length of the walks and have now started using the exercise bike again. I have noticed that, by the end of a walk, my fingers are usually swollen but I don't know the reason why. I suppose some fluid must be building up somewhere. Depending on individual circumstances, it takes people three to six months to return to their normal level of activity. What I have found difficulty accepting is my body needs both time and energy to recover and heal. It also needs rest, something I am not good at.

Monday 8
The birth of The Coffee Club! I spent the morning with two close friends from school – Liz was going into hospital this afternoon for an operation, Sue was on maternity leave and about to deliver her second child any time. They were the ones facing the delights (?) of a hospital stay but it was my hands that were cold. I will never really understand my body.

Tuesday 9
The second time on the golf course with Kate, my "guardian physiotherapist" and we played eleven holes – I forgot to mention to her that the consultant had said a maximum of nine holes to begin with. Today was the first time I had worn a bra since the lumpectomy and it felt rather strange being confined again. We stayed for the traditional Ladies' Christmas Lunch and as the coffee and mints arrived I began to feel distinctly unwell. I had not consumed any alcohol as I had the car and the food had tasted fine. By the time I arrived home I had a blinding headache and the scar under the arm was so hot I

could have fried an egg on it! I slept on the settee for a couple of hours but felt very light-headed when I woke up. I have no idea what my temperature was but the central heating had to be turned off! Most unusually for me, I gave in and went to bed.

The baby, a girl, was born this morning.

Wednesday 10
Having slept for nearly twelve hours I woke up covered in sweat and, after a shower, decided it would be a good idea to ring the surgery for an appointment. The scar felt quite tender, looked rather fierce and was still very hot to the touch. However, my doctor was not due to be on duty and I did not want to see anyone else. I spent the day indoors and took a Nurofen tablet every four hours.

The professional at the golf club organises a quiz once a year and I didn't want to let our partners down. I am glad we made the effort to go tonight because we won a spot prize of a huge tin of Quality Street.

Thursday 11
A trip to the doctor's, an infection in the wound was diagnosed and antibiotics were prescribed – more tablets to swallow. Great! I am a loose woman again because I think the infection was the result of my bra rubbing against the scar when I played golf on Tuesday.

Friday 12
Already the antibiotics are beginning to take effect as the scar seems a bit cooler and so do I; the central heating has been turned on again. John's office Christmas Dinner was tonight and never before has the phrase "I have nothing to wear" been so appropriate. However, we had already decided we would not be attending this year. At least I have another twelve months to sort out an outfit for next December!

Monday 15
Now home after her operation I visited Liz, the senior member of the Coffee Club, to offer my expert advice on the art of recuperation. This mainly consisted of drinking cups of tea and three games of Scrabble! At least it was a fairer contest than playing the computer even though I lost two games to one.

Tuesday 16
A second Christmas lunch for me this year as wives were invited to attend the Rotary Club meeting. After the problems of last week's lunch I made sure I left my bra in the airing cupboard and wore a fairly loose fitting top.

One of the targets I set myself before the operation was to be fit enough to attend the school's Carol Service. For reasons I cannot really explain, even to myself, it was important I was there. I sat at the back of the church next to a parent who had lost her husband to cancer almost a year ago. At Parents' Consultation Evenings there was always plenty of good-natured banter with them and in-between we discussed the progress made by their children. By the end of the service we were both feeling pretty emotional.

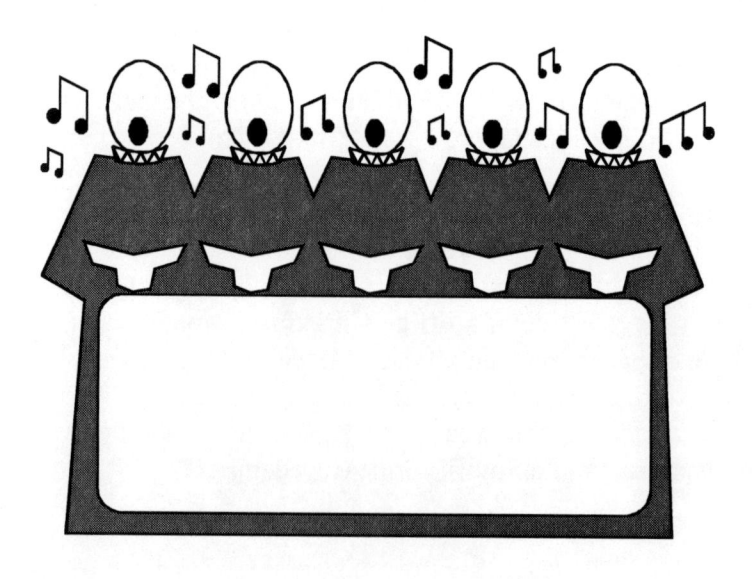

Neighbours: Steph and Max kiss for the first time since the chemotherapy began.

Wednesday 17
I went into school this morning to help with the final dancing session before the Year 11 Ball tomorrow night. It was good to return to familiar surroundings and the students seemed genuinely pleased to see me. Many were very direct in the questions they asked about the operation and what was going to happen next. That's the beauty of working with kids – no frills, usually they cut straight to the chase.

Eventually I managed to leave the building and went to collect one third of the Coffee Club as we had an important little person and her mother to visit. The Coffee Club has grown to three point five.

Thursday 18
It never ceases to amaze the staff how, within the space of a few hours, Year 11 leave school in their uniform and return later in the evening looking ten years older and very sophisticated. Many of the students had pooled their resources and arrived in stretch limousines. Elegant ball gowns and dinner jackets everywhere, flowers and presents were exchanged, cameras flashed to record the event for posterity. The dancing lessons paid dividends as the students expertly waltzed, performed the veleta, Cumberland Eight, barn dance and Spanish Swing. As always, the traditional Candlelit Supper stole the show. The Drama Studio had been converted for one night only into a candlelit restaurant offering a large finger buffet – sandwiches, chicken pieces, pizza pieces, cheese and pineapple on sticks, dips, crisps, chocolate logs and the obligatory sausages on sticks. The recipe for the punch has remained a closely guarded secret from the students for over three decades. The Ball has always been one of the highlights in the school year and this one was no exception. Another target achieved.

Friday 19
I had a shock this morning – I started another period and it is only twelve days since the previous one finished. If there is such a thing as reincarnation I want to place on record my wish to return as a man!

Sunday 21
The Outlaw's birthday and John's sister had organised a family lunch at a local pub. We had a pleasant meal and were able to catch up on all the gossip.

Monday 22
Radiotherapy
Radiotherapy (or radiation therapy) uses high-energy rays, usually x-rays, both to treat cancer and to reduce the risk of the cancer returning. These rays are produced by a machine called a linear accelerator and are able to damage and destroy any remaining cancer cells within the treatment area. However, the rays also affect normal cells in the area being treated. For the treatment planning a special x-ray machine called a simulator is used. It moves in exactly the same way as the linear accelerator but, instead of giving treatment, it takes x-rays to help the radiographer plan the correct position for "zapping" the patient.

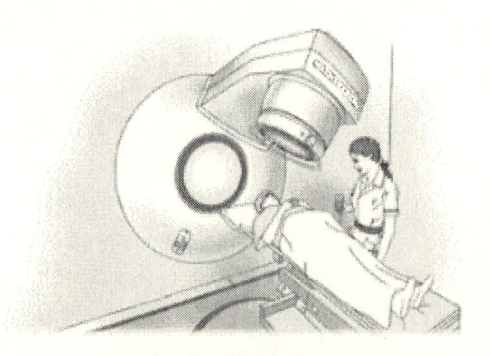

First Visit to the Bristol Royal Infirmary
Today was nothing short of a personal waking nightmare and I definitely do not want to return to the hospital once let alone

twenty-five times. Because the oncologist was unavoidably delayed I was waiting in the radiography room for fifteen minutes on my own with just the huge machine to stare at. At the back of the room were several shelves full of Perspex masks. They triggered memories of watching the serialisation of "The Man in the Iron Mask" on television. I remembered thinking at the time how barbaric it was to enclose a person's head in that way. These masks looked very claustrophobic to me and I almost freaked at the thought I might have to wear one of them.

The oncologist arrived and drew some lines on my skin to indicate where the tumour had been. The radiographers then positioned me on the couch under the simulator and took an outline of my body. One of them joked that the reason for this was to measure how much weight I put on over Christmas! Unfortunately, I was feeling so scared that I didn't really appreciate her attempt at being humorous. With my upper body resting against a wedge the "T" bar was lowered until it was just above my head. My hands grasped the ends of the bar and the radiographers then moved my arms until the elbows were pointing towards the respective walls at the sides of the room. Lying on the couch with both my arms making right angles, my neck was rotated almost 90^0 away from the affected right breast. My instructions were to lie motionless in this fixed position for nearly thirty minutes whilst various measurements and x-rays were taken. These, together with the body outline, were transferred to the planning computers so that the most effective dose of radiation could be calculated and, once the exact area of treatment was finalised, my skin was marked up. I had three separate pinpricks of permanent ink tattoos that the radiographers will use to line up the beams when the treatment starts next month. I think the needle that marked the right side of the breast touched either a nerve or scar tissue because it was painful to say the least and I nearly jumped off the couch. It was a huge relief when I could, at last, put my arms down and look in front of me instead of to the left. The arms were fine but my neck felt stiff and I had a thumping headache – probably the result of tension.

During the last three or four days I have had to dig really deep inside and am feeling very scared and vulnerable.

Tuesday 23
My period finished – I have never had one last only four days before. Thinking back to the conversation with the breast care sister, she did suggest I might be pre-menopausal. So, am I still pre-menopausal or menopausal?

Wednesday 24
With the Christmas presents loaded in the car, we drove up to Surrey to spend a few days with my family.

Thursday 25
Opened the presents from John and my parents before going to Sarah and James's for lunch. It was the first time I had seen her since breaking the news and we were both conscious of the fact that only our husbands knew what had been going on. With other people constantly around much remained unspoken but, in a strange sisterly way, much was said between us. So different from when she was four and, in a fit of temper, tried to push me onto the open log fire. And then there was the time she locked me in a wardrobe. Oh, and once set fire to my doll's pram. Sisters – who needs them? Me. I couldn't have coped without her.

I had to turn down the usual game of football with my nephews and be careful that my niece, who was rather excited, didn't bump into me. After a late lunch we settled down to playing some games and I must admit the "little kids" (although one nephew is only fourteen and at least four inches taller than his aunt) displayed more patience waiting to open their presents than this particular "big kid". There again this Christmas was a bonus for me and another tick to go on my checklist of targets to achieve.

Saturday 27
The annual "pilgrimage" to the Bentall Centre and certain other selected shops in Kingston-upon-Thames for the sales. January sales in December and yes, we did spot Easter eggs in several shops. I didn't buy anything but John bought a new suit and some shirts for work.

Sunday 28
As usual we brought back more than we took with us! We had a really good Christmas but it is nice to be home and not have to keep up the deception. However, I strongly suspect that I wasn't the only family member wearing a mask at times. What price family secrets? I guess it must be hereditary that we all try desperately to protect each other.

Monday 29
John is struggling with a very bad cold and coughed so hard today that he burst blood vessels around his eyes and forehead. I am desperately trying to avoid catching it with Tuesday 6 January looming large on the horizon, although any excuse not to return to the BRI again would be brilliant. I am not looking forward to this radiotherapy lark one little bit and wish there was a way round it. On the other hand, to have to face chemotherapy would be a horrendous ordeal for me so why am I moaning?

Tuesday 30
We decided some exercise and fresh air might revive us after the festivities. For the first time since early October we played golf together and managed ten holes. The bra of course remained at home!

Wednesday 31
The deal was I would watch the Lord of the Ring films with John if he came to see the Harry Potter films with me. This afternoon we went to see the last film of the trilogy, Return of the King. Towards the end of the marathon film I felt

decidedly uncomfortable with stomach cramps. I was sweating one minute and almost shivering the next. When we arrived home I went straight to bed and slept for two hours. Later on I passed some blood and posters I have seen recently about bowel cancer immediately came to mind. OK, Jeeves, I think it is time for us to go surfing some different websites.

Dear God,
It's Mamma Gram; can I interrupt you for half a minute? Just now I am terrified at the prospect of having a different form of cancer. I'm not sure whether this is yet another test of my resolve – if it is please give me the strength and courage to pull through.

Whilst at college, a friend gave me a bookmark with the first eight lines of Charlotte Bronte's poem "Life" on it. I used to read it every day during my final teaching practice at a secondary school in a socially deprived area in South Yorkshire. Somehow the sentiments seem appropriate again.

Life, believe, is not a dream
So dark as sages say;
Oft a little morning rain
Foretells a pleasant day.
Sometimes there are clouds of gloom,
But these are transient all;
If the shower will make the roses bloom,
O why lament its fall?

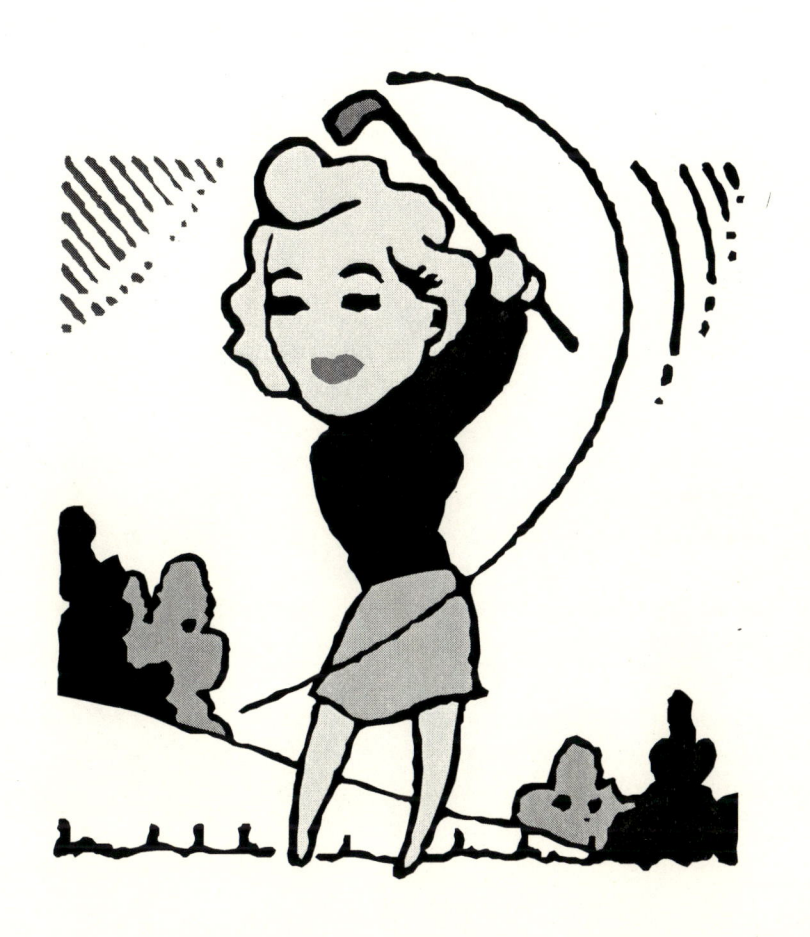

"In golf as in life it is the follow through that makes the difference."

January 2004

Monday 5
Having put off my smear test last August because of everything else that was going on, my appointment was today. Great timing to have it the day before the radiotherapy starts but, if I hadn't gone, I would have kept finding excuses to avoid it. Needless to say I dreaded the test more than usual – I have had one brush with cancer and am scared about the possibility of bowel cancer although I cannot tell anybody else of my fears at the moment. In for a penny, in for a pound, I asked the nurse to do a cholesterol blood test, something else I had been putting off for months even though my mother and sister both have problems.

This evening I marked up the calendar in the hall with a countdown from twenty-five to one so that I can cross off a number each day when I return home from the treatment. John had printed information sheets on twenty-four members of the Spurs squad as another countdown for me – the twenty-fifth "member" is to be a special surprise.

Neighbours: Steph is offended at Izzy's suggestion to wear some of her old wigs.

Tuesday 6
No. 25 – Bobby Zamora
Let zapping commence!
The first four radiotherapy sessions are scheduled for three o'clock. As the senior member of the Coffee Club knows

about my hospital phobia only too well, Liz invited me to spend the "waiting time" with her rather than sit at home alone worrying. Although I feel perfectly well I am not allowed to drive the daily one hundred mile round trip myself. John was today's chauffeur and friends at the golf club have organised a rota to help out. I am really grateful for their kindness and support but, being a fiercely independent person, feel I am imposing on people and their time. Added to which I prefer to drive than be driven!

No prizes for guessing my physical state as the nervous system took control around midday. I was offered lunch but couldn't eat anything. The chauffeur arrived just before half past one to whisk me away. Recognising my "symptoms" he switched on Radio 2 and, as we drove to Bristol, I decided to keep a daily record of the number of Eddie Stobart lorries spotted. Sad – I need to get out more! Instinctively I knew I needed to focus on something totally stupid.

I checked in at reception and sat down as requested to wait for my name to be called to go down to the basement where the oncology department is situated. A man sitting opposite me had a scar round his neck. He was telling his friend about the mask he has to wear to keep his head still during the radiotherapy treatment. So now I know who and what the masks are for – I wish I had been told two weeks ago. I heard my name and we walked towards the lift.

Before the first zapping a senior radiographer took me into a consulting room to talk about caring for myself during the treatment. I was advised to eat a well-balanced, healthy diet, drink plenty of water and listen to my body regarding taking a rest during the day. Wearing soft cotton tops to avoid rubbing the skin was recommended and I might feel more comfortable without a bra. (No arguments there, I have been a loose woman for several weeks!) As I have permanent tattoos I can shower as normal but must not use any perfumed soap or shampoo and it was suggested that I used my hands rather than a flannel to wash the breast and armpit. (No problems, I never use a flannel in the shower.) Finally, I was given a tube of aqueous cream to rub onto the breast to keep it hydrated. She reassured me by saying the treatment would not make me radioactive so it was perfectly safe to mix with and touch other people! I guess that is a radiographer's standard joke. However, on a more serious note, I needed to be aware that the radiotherapy normally takes two weeks to become effective so five weeks treatment would be seven weeks in reality.

We then went down the corridor to SL755A a number I would become familiar with – my treatment room. As we turned the corner there was the proper machine looking like a huge telephone receiver and as large as the dummy one I endured two weeks ago. I was asked to remove my top and lie on the couch. The bar came down and I took hold of it as in the planning session. The two radiographers then referred to the computer and positioned the machine and me in exactly the right place. Before leaving the room they explained that they would be watching me carefully on CCTV in case I needed anything. A button was pushed and the room was plunged into semi-darkness; after a few seconds the machine started making a noise – the zaps had begun. I was concentrating so hard on remaining motionless that I forgot to breathe! Music playing from a cassette recorder was not loud enough to drown out the sound of the linear accelerator. I began counting the seconds until the noise stopped.

One of the radiographers returned to change the angle of the machine for the second dose of x-rays. We went through the same procedure as before – press button, leave room, lights off, noise and zappo. Oh boy, I started counting again, tried to relax and breathe normally. I honestly thought that the lumpectomy was going to be harder to deal with than the radiotherapy – did I ever make such a wrong judgement. Heaven knows how I am going to face another twenty-four sessions.

The noise eventually stopped again and as the radiographer entered the room she told me to relax and let go of the bar. She came over to the couch, moved the bar and head of the machine out of the way and said I could now get dressed. I didn't need telling twice; no bra to bother with so the rugby shirt went on in double-quick time while my appointment sheet was initialled. I almost ran down the corridor to the waiting area, grabbed my husband by the arm and headed straight to the lift. Beam me up, Scotty, and make it quick!

On the way home we stopped to buy some baby soap and shampoo. After I showered tonight I rubbed some of the aqueous cream onto the skin. I now know exactly where the lump was as I feel quite tender and need to take care not to rub so hard in future.
(4 Stobarts)

Wednesday 7
No. 24 – Rob Burch
John was chauffeur again and the parasympathetic nervous system was working overtime even by my standards. It is my intention to ask the radiographers to give me the remaining twenty-three zaps in one go tomorrow otherwise I am going to do something stupid like not turn up for the appointments. I emailed Simon and asked him for whatever the next stage is after prayers and miracles. I also desperately need some sleep to recharge the batteries.
(3 Stobarts)

Thursday 8
No. 23 – Christian Ziege
I had my hair cut this morning and the hairdresser remarked that I had a couple of thin patches of hair around the hairline. She knows about the cancer and promised to tell me if she was concerned about anything.

A letter arrived from my doctor to tell me that my cholesterol was measured at 7.7, which is considered to be high, and that he wanted to prescribe atorvastatins. MORE TABLETS!

Today it was the turn of Kate to play chauffeur. Having someone who knew my medical phobia really well was a great help because I could be myself instead of putting on a show of bravado. After two days of driving to Bristol in glorious sunshine the weather was absolutely awful, windy, bucketing with rain, spray being thrown up by lorries and I wished it was me behind the wheel – not because I didn't trust her, I just felt it was unfair and an imposition. When I tried to explain this and apologise, Kate told me that it was both a relief and important for other people to feel they were actually involved in doing something tangible and not merely stuck on the periphery sending me cards or flowers, lending books or jigsaw puzzles to relieve my boredom. I knew exactly what she meant – if roles were reversed I would happily have been playing chauffeur for her every day or doing anything else to help for that matter – but still I felt tremendously guilty. I guess it is hard for me to accept that people care.

For the record I bottled asking the radiographers for the remaining treatments to be given in one go.
(5 Stobarts)

Friday 9
No. 22 – Rohan Ricketts
It poured with rain again today. An ex-colleague and close friend had the dubious "pleasure" of coping with this particular phobic but again it was important I felt comfortable with someone other than John in the first week of treatment. While we were waiting in the basement a young man approached, apologised for interrupting and addressed me by my name. My initial thought was my luck had changed and I had a male radiographer to look after me! Stand aside, George Clooney, your days are definitely numbered. Then common sense prevailed as he introduced himself. Due to a different hairstyle and hair colour, plus the fact he was fifteen years older than last time we met, I had failed to recognise an ex-student from school. We had time to catch up on the intervening years, including his training as a psychiatric nurse (he always was three cans short of a six-pack at school so it seemed appropriate) before he told us that his father had lung

cancer and emphysema and had been given one month to live. They were at the hospital so his father could have radiotherapy in an attempt to lessen his considerable pain. I looked across to the man lying on a trolley and coughing painfully. He was a shadow of his former self. Certain types of cancer can do that to people.

I have no real recollection of today's treatment – as I lay on the couch, I thought about "Westy's" father and said a few silent prayers for him.
(3 Stobarts)

Saturday 10
The first of two days off for good behaviour! Yesterday's chauffeur and his wife had invited us round for a meal. By the way, they were the couple that led me astray and took me horseracing last November.

Monday 12
No. 21 – Mbulelo Mabizela
A most unexpected start to the week as I had a phone call from the Head of PE at school to let me know I was Manager of the Week in the Schools Fantasy Football League. I had accumulated 32 points and a certificate was on its way! As he, like two of my nephews and their father, is a Chelsea supporter, I took great delight ribbing him that a FEMALE SPURS FAN had beaten all the male staff.

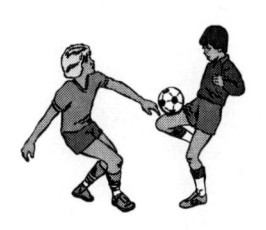

My treatment time has moved forward to twenty past two just for today. Today's chauffeur was Nicky, a friend from the golf club who had breast cancer two years ago and so had been there, done that and bought the T-shirts. She had

rung me before Christmas and offered to answer any questions I might have regarding the radiotherapy treatment. The zaps were delayed twenty minutes and I was glad she was there to keep me relatively sane. It must have been a strange experience for her to be there in a different capacity. I am not entirely sure but the noise from the machine seemed to come in different bursts today.
(9 Stobarts)

Neighbours: Steph is feeling smothered by the attention she is receiving from Max and her father.

Tuesday 13
No. 20 – Jonathan Blondel
The Coffee Club reconvened in full for the first time this year. When John arrived to collect me I had my hands full rocking Point Five to sleep. I was pleased that all my years of training with five nephews and one niece had not deserted me. Just over four weeks old, she looked the picture of contentment with not a care in the world. I hoped that holding the baby at such a delicate stage of falling asleep would be a valid excuse not to go for treatment – so much for wishful thinking.

My appointment time has changed yet again to two o'clock. I was under the impression that appointments would be given at a similar time each day so that I could establish a routine for eating, resting etc. Now I am sitting in the waiting area with a different group of people and hearing about other forms of cancer. One thing is absolutely certain – the more I hear the luckier I feel. In many respects I was fortunate to find the lump early, to be registered with a brilliant GP who never wastes a second of time, and to be diagnosed with what is generally regarded as one of the more "treatable" cancers with a high rate of survival. I have much to be thankful for but, nevertheless, some days have been very dark deep inside me and the mask has worked overtime. I can't recall seeing my name on the list of Oscar nominations.
(10 Stobarts)

Wednesday 14
No. 19 – Dean Richards
I saw someone from the golf club in the lower waiting area – he is driving his wife to the hospital every day for treatment on her leg. Unfortunately this is her second battle with the disease. When I arrived at ten to two he said there had been a power cut in the morning, her appointment should have been at twenty to one and she had only just gone in! You can imagine how I felt but, five minutes later, my name was called. Relief or what? However, on the way home I felt some stinging and was uncomfortable at times during the evening so I applied the aqueous cream twice.

The best part of today was the whole process took only two and a half hours. I was picked up at half past twelve and was back home putting the kettle on for coffee at three o'clock. For once the motorway was fairly clear and the traffic in the Clifton area of Bristol was free flowing. As far as I am concerned, I hope this trend continues through to the last session.
(7 Stobarts)

Thursday 15
No. 18 – Milenko Acimovic
This morning in W H Smith's a woman came up to me and asked if I was Mamma Gram. She is a supply teacher and has worked at school in the distant past. She explained she was recovering from breast cancer and thought she had seen me a few weeks ago at the BRI. We stood by the birthday cards and exchanged notes on our respective progress. As today was her first radiotherapy session I was able to explain what would happen and put her mind at rest. I actually felt I had done something useful for a change.

Anne insisted on parking on the top level of the multi-storey car park so that I could enjoy the view over Bristol. However, the wind was blowing a gale so the sightseeing was cut short by mutual consent!

At the hospital I saw a little girl aged about four or five expertly manoeuvring around in a wheelchair. It was obvious that she had undergone chemotherapy as she had lost all her hair. She refused to allow her father to push her around and appeared to have a real sense of independence and determination.
(3 Stobarts)

Friday 16
No. 17 – Anthony Gardner
At a golf club function this evening I was asked to talk to a member's wife about the effects of having radiotherapy. Because her lump had been near a lung, she would be having thirty treatments. It was another chance for me to help by doing something constructive rather than sit on the periphery.
(3 Stobarts)

Saturday 17
Another two days of respite from the zaps of that wonderful machine. Spurs beat Liverpool 2-1 and I could not resist the urge to send Liz a gloating email.
Whilst applying the aqueous cream after a shower, I noticed a "bruise" on the skin above the breast scar that appeared to be the shape and size of the lump. The breast definitely feels harder than the other one at the moment – I suppose it is a build-up of scar tissue.

Sunday 18
We spent some time looking for a new white gas cooker and visited the usual retailers. Basically we just want to replace like for like. A fairly straightforward task one would think especially as we don't want anything too fancy. Wrong! There were loads of stainless steel cookers to choose from but who in their right mind wants one of those? You spend most of your time wiping the surface to remove various marks. I wonder who conducted the market research on cookers? If only they had asked me for my opinion! Anyway, after

searching around we were left with the choice of either buying a particular cooker or not buying it. We decided to return home and investigate other options on the Internet.

Monday 19
No. 16 – Ledley King
Why does the weekend pass so quickly? I felt very fragile first thing this morning and just couldn't stop crying. I remembered what the breast care sister had told me about giving in to my emotions and being kind to myself but I simply didn't know what had triggered this intense outburst. Everyone keeps telling me how much he or she admires the manner in which I have tackled this cancer business and commented on how strong I must be physically and mentally. Perhaps I should receive an Oscar for fooling people into thinking I am handling the situation better than in reality. Fortunately Nicky was driving so I didn't have to pretend that everything in my world was fine.

The treatment time has moved forward to ten to one – at least I now have eleven sessions at this earlier time and have adjusted my routine accordingly.
(6 Stobarts)

Tuesday 20
No. 15 – Jamie Redknapp
After feeling so low yesterday, the last thing I needed today was a thirty-minute wait for the zaps. As the machine spewed out its x-rays I tried to imagine I was lying on a sunny, sandy beach thousands of miles away. It wasn't really that difficult because it was (a) where I wanted to be – in a little corner of the world completely on my own – and (b) the music playing was a Beach Boys' CD.

Being a mathematics teacher, I have tried to reflect logically on the emotional roller coaster of the past two days. In spite of what the medical staff have said, in spite of the material I have read, in spite of the incredible and overwhelming support from family and friends, such is the unpredictability of cancer that a part of me is absolutely petrified the disease could return any time and anywhere in my body. It takes much energy to push these dark, negative thoughts out of my mind but the stark truth is **I have had cancer** and, whether I like it or not, it has changed my life. To what extent I cannot say at this stage but I suppose I have been given an opportunity to re-evaluate my priorities.

I honestly don't know how much the cancer has affected John's life. Typical man, he doesn't talk much about it but has been incredibly supportive in his usual quiet way.
(10 Stobarts)

Wednesday 21
No. 14 – Gustavo Poyet
Today's delay was the worst so far – an hour and twenty minutes. The couple that had driven me to the hospital had gone shopping down the road in Broadmead and I had no way of contacting them to explain my predicament. As I sat in the waiting area I became more and more anxious and frustrated. I hate having my time wasted unnecessarily and do not like doing it to other people especially when they are giving up a large part of their day for me. After the treatment I literally ran all the way to the multi-storey car park. I was quite pleased I managed to do it – I must be fitter than I thought. I apologised for the inconvenience but they appeared less concerned about it all than I was!

Although my breast is beginning to look red I don't feel any soreness. Perhaps the years of sunbathing have toughened my skin.
(3 Stobarts)

Thursday 22
No. 13 – Kasey Keller
Courtesy of a national newspaper we had amassed a stack of CDs so I decided to donate them to the hospital. Having seen only eight CDs in the treatment room I thought they would be going to a good home! After today's treatment I have crossed

the halfway point so it is downhill from now on, thank goodness.
(8 Stobarts)

Friday 23
No. 12 – Gary Doherty
After a thirty-five-minute delay yesterday I was called in on time today! As I walked into the room I glanced at the display screen attached to the wall and thought there was something different about it. I did not recognise the colouring or the numbers; I looked at the top of the screen and read my surname but a different first name. Um, excuse me, I am the other Mrs Gram – please can I have my own zaps?

The scar on the breast is beginning to turn white on one side but the one under the armpit is still quite pink. The areola on my right breast appears to be changing colour and is quite misshapen, I would say almost puckered in towards the nipple in places. It is also smoother than before the operation and the nipple is completely inverted. The third "scar" is still quite obvious as a ridge and shows no sign of disappearing.
(8 Stobarts)

Saturday 24
Yet another weekend off, the staff at the hospital must really like me! Either that or they want some R and R time. Having witnessed firsthand how hard they work and admired their professionalism, they deserve to indulge themselves.

Sunday 25
Spurs FA Cup fourth round away tie at Manchester City was shown live on TV and finished as a one-all draw. The weather forecast was predicting snow blizzards. I managed to complete forty minutes on the exercise bike today.

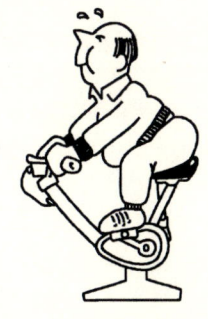

Monday 26
No. 11 – Stephane Dalmat
Before today's treatment I was unexpectedly taken to an examination room for an ultrasound scan. Immediately my mind raced back to the terrifying emotions associated with the previous scan in October and, accordingly, the stomach performed a perfect triple somersault with a double twist thrown in for good measure. I clenched my fists as the probe moved painfully across my still very tender breast and, eventually, plucked up the courage to glance at the display screen on my right. From memory the image looked different from last time and, even to my untrained eyes, appeared clear. The radiographer would not make specific comments on the image she was looking at but explained that it would be used to calculate the precise area and dosage of the booster treatment.
(5 Stobarts)

Tuesday 27
No. 10 – Robbie Keane
As I lay on the couch my two radiographers were bemoaning the fact that the snow hadn't been heavy enough to prevent them from coming to work today. I decided to draw their attention to this particular patient's thoughts about snowfalls at this particular time in her life! Apart from anything else I had been told it was important that my treatment continued as planned and I did not miss any appointments.

On the journey home we stopped at a golf club and I bought a waterproof suit and a wolf head cover for my driver in the sales – a present to myself for managing to make it this far, an incentive to keep going and, most importantly, a bargain my mum would have been proud of. As Simon has been trying hard to persuade me to do something indulgent for several months, I might score some points and he might forget to use the "I" word for a while!
(3 Stobarts)

Wednesday 28
No. 9 – Fredi Kanoute
Typical – the couple who had to wait nearly an hour and a half for me were delayed again! At least they were prepared for it – books to read, a thermos flask, a blanket. To date only one treatment has been at the appointment time whereas Nicky told me that nearly all her treatments were on time. I heard today that the radiotherapy machines are in constant use from eight in the morning until eight at night. Goodness knows how many patients are zapped every day – in many respects the hospital is like a production line. I sincerely hope that all the "end products" pass the quality control tests.
(4 Stobarts)

Thursday 29
No. 8 – Helder Postiga
My machine was broken and so I had to transfer to one in a room with an "F" code at the other end of the corridor. Variety is the spice of life and the walk made a pleasant change to the normal routine!

For the first time since the treatment started I actually felt physically tired and mentally shattered. It was virtually impossible to concentrate on anything and all I wanted to do was shut the world out and drift away to a deserted island. I couldn't even find the words to talk to Simon about my low mood and felt guilty for wasting his valuable time. However, as I had been invited out for an evening meal with friends I had to put the mask in place and try hard to stay awake and make polite conversation.
(4 Stobarts)

Friday 30
No. 7 – Darren Anderton
One of the senior radiographers came to tell me that the ultrasound scan I had on Monday was clear, which was a huge relief, and then she explained about the procedure for the booster treatment. Unfortunately she could not show me the

treatment room as it was in use all day so, next Tuesday, I will be stepping into the unknown again which is rather scary to say the least.

During this afternoon's treatment the staff changed halfway through. Now, after eighteen sessions, I know the procedure inside and out, forwards and backwards, so I did not appreciate the overly pedantic radiographer who entered the room at the end of my zaps and told me when and exactly how to move off the couch!

When I arrived home from the hospital, I reread all the Get Well cards and letters and played my All Time Classic Tearjerkers CD. Something somewhere deep inside appeared to be urging me to protect myself. That probably sounds crazy but I suspect my body was telling me to drop the mask and put my own needs first for once in my life.
(4 Stobarts)

Saturday 31
A headline which appeared today in one of the national daily newspapers: "Cider county is hit by a quake".

Apparently at half past six last Thursday night the town where we live experienced a minor earthquake that measured 3.1 on the Richter scale. A small movement in a fault line in the Earth generally causes Earth tremors and there are many fault lines throughout the southwest of England.

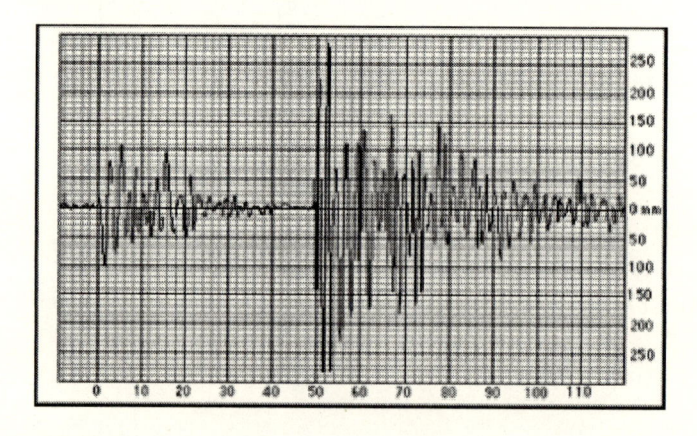

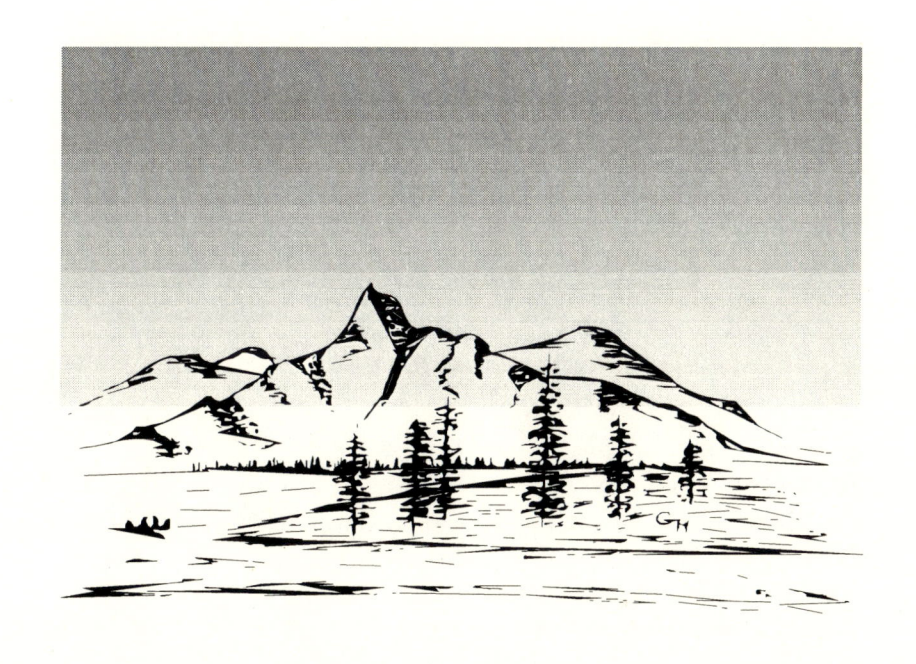

"There are many paths to the top of the mountain but the view is always the same."

February

Sunday 1
The search for a white gas cooker has not been very successful so it was back to Currys to place an order for the choice of one from one!

I pedalled for forty-five minutes on the exercise bike this afternoon, as it was too windy to go out on my proper bike.

Monday 2
No. 6 – Simon Davies
The traffic news on the radio warned that road works on the motorway were causing thirty-five to forty minute delays and the Clifton Suspension Bridge was closed because of the Fathers 4 Justice protesters. I rang Pauline to tell her about the impending problems and asked if she could pick me up earlier than arranged. As a result we had to use the A38 and then find another way into the City Centre. Interesting to say the least as neither of us really knew our way around Bristol. A combination of skilful driving and remarkable navigation i.e. the ability to quickly read signposts meant we arrived at the hospital in plenty of time only to discover a twenty-five minute delay for treatment!

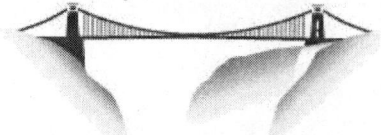

CLIFTONSUSPENSIONBRIDGE

A boost is when the x-rays are directed to the actual area where the lump was. Before today's radiotherapy I was marked up for the booster treatment. Unlike the treatment planning session in December, temporary ink markings were used to draw a rectangle on my skin. I was told to be careful not to rub them off in the shower so it is back to imitating a contortionist again.

One of the radiographers joked I should be able to give her a rest and quote the machine settings myself as I had heard them nineteen times already. No thanks – I'd prefer to leave the responsibility to the professional.
(3 Stobarts)

Tuesday 3
No. 5 – Goran Bunjevcevic
Last evening's news bulletin gave out that the men on the bridge had enough provisions for a week so John allowed two hours to drive to the hospital. Lo and behold, no road works, the protesters had been arrested so the bridge was reopened and we were fifty minutes early for my twelve-thirty appointment. I spy ……….!

The booster treatment was in room SL22B and I had the luxury of lying down flat on the couch, resting my head on a pillow and keeping my arms by my side. What a change from being propped up by a wedge and holding onto the bar above my head. The downside, which was nothing really, was the machine was positioned closer to my body.
(2 Stobarts)

Wednesday 4
No. 4 – Kazuyuki Toda
As I waited in the main corridor another patient asked me how I was coping with the treatment. I replied I was fine and had been fortunate not to experience any real side effects. She, on the other hand, had been very tired and the skin on her breast was red and itching.
(3 Stobarts)

Before my first treatment I was told that my body would use much energy over the course of twenty-five radiotherapy sessions. I am supposed to be conserving my energy and resting as necessary so what did I do tonight? Only subject my body to the traumas of watching Spurs play Manchester City in the FA Cup fourth round replay. Three-nil to the good at half time and Spurs were cruising; the so-called experts said the match was all over bar the shouting. However, City had other ideas and came out for the second half like a team possessed – or one that had received some words of "encouragement" from the manager. During the post-match analysis the experts did a U-turn and called it one of the greatest ever comebacks as City won by four goals to three in stoppage time. Being philosophical I suppose it was long-awaited sweet revenge for their defeat in the 1981 FA Cup Final replay when Spurs' Ricky Villa scored the best ever goal in a cup final, not that I am biased.

Thursday 5
No. 3 – Mauricio Taricco
Today I talked to a man suffering from throat and stomach cancer. He had not eaten or tasted proper food since August and had to take his nourishment intravenously.
(2 Stobarts)

Friday 6
No. 2 – Stephen Carr
The penultimate session and my "guardian physiotherapist" had insisted on chauffeuring one more time. Kate commented that I appeared to be more relaxed than the first time she drove me to Bristol. However, one touch of my ice-cold hand quickly reassured her that everything was normal for me!

I talked to a senior radiographer about the forthcoming holiday to Tenerife and was advised to keep the skin in the treatment area covered at all times and to regularly apply a sun block with a protection factor of at least 15. The only time I use sun cream is to act as a moisturising layer between my

skin and the bug repellent spray when on holiday in the States. Tamoxifen tablets, pyjama shirts and shorts, a dressing gown, baby soap and shampoo, aqueous cream, sun cream – what next? This cancer lark is, most definitely, an expensive business!
(9 Stobarts)

Saturday 7
Not having hit a golf ball for nearly six weeks I thought it would be a good idea to spend some time on the practice area and try to gradually re-educate the muscles.

Sunday 8
Fortunately we were at home most of the day because the new cooker was delivered!

Monday 9
No. 1 – The Official History of Tottenham Hotspur Football Club DVD
LAST DAY!
I never thought this day would arrive and, typically, we encountered a problem. A lorry had knocked down the traffic lights at a major crossroads on the outskirts of town and a diversion was in place. Bumper to bumper, stop, start, it took over half an hour to reach the motorway junction.

As I checked in at level B, the receptionist knew it was my final treatment and she wished me good luck for the future. I felt really touched and thanked her. All the members of staff at the hospital have been fantastic.

Although the treatment finished today there was a two-week delay in the x-rays kicking in so I will be "radioactive" for another fortnight! The permanent tattoos mean I cannot have radiotherapy in that area again. John and I celebrated my "silver zap" by having lunch at a restaurant in Bristol and a bottle of bubbly with dinner. Indulgent twice in one day – Simon will never believe it!
(7 Stobarts)

Tuesday 10
Luxury – I am a free agent and the days are mine to control again. So why does it feel a huge anticlimax? I should be doing "Robbie Keane somersaults" in celebration; instead I have to adjust to another new routine.

I calculated that I travelled over 2660 miles between home and the hospital, crossed the Clifton Suspension Bridge fifty times (should have been fifty-two) for a total cost of £15 in toll charges and counted 128 Eddie Stobart lorries. Sad or what? The Office Staff at school described me as a typical mathematics teacher, always counting.

To acknowledge my radiotherapy "stayability" the Coffee Club treated me to lunch. As we sat at the table I counted 13 Stobarts! Once a Stobart counter, always a Stobart counter.

Wednesday 11
As the sun was shining and with the holiday fast approaching, I decided to spend an hour at the golf club and hit some golf balls on the practice area.

Thursday 12
One of the breast care sisters at our local hospital rang me this morning to find out how I had coped with the radiotherapy. She asked if I was feeling tired and whether I had experienced any problems with my skin burning or peeling. I said I was fine, just very relieved the five weeks of treatment were finally over. Although I will have regular check-ups with the oncologist and consultant surgeon, she reassured me that if I had any concerns at all, no matter how trivial they might seem, to contact the breast care unit rather than sit worrying at home.

I had my usual pre-holiday hair cut this afternoon and the hairdresser said she was surprised it was in such good condition given the treatment only finished on Monday. My hair does not appear to be quite as thick as before the cancer was diagnosed but, on the other hand, it is not falling out in large handfuls.

Friday 13
My first real test of stamina as I drove the 150 miles to my parents' house in Surrey. Apart from the right arm feeling a bit stiff and tingly I didn't experience any problems, another positive step forward in the recovery process.

Saturday 14
We were up early to drive to London Gatwick Airport. Never one to do mornings well, I wasn't really thinking (no change there then!) and went to lift my golf bag into the car. Rather like forgetting the drainage bottles in hospital three months ago, not a mistake to make a second time.

The flight to Tenerife lasted about four hours and, in spite of the warnings about deep vein thrombosis, I could not face the thought of wearing those wretched surgical stockings. Instead I tried performing some of the recommended long-haul flight exercises. In the absence of any in-flight entertainment they did at least relieve some of the boredom and increase my contortionist skills.

Sunday 15
Our first round of golf was at Las Americas and, not having played eighteen holes since early October, I was pleased to survive in one piece especially as I had worn a bra! The fact that the sun was shining and the temperature was 72°F probably helped to keep the muscles warm and me fairly relaxed. I have always been a hothouse plant.

This afternoon the water in the hotel swimming pool came nowhere near passing the toe test. Even John said it was too cold and he doesn't usually forego a swim. As sunbathing was out of the question because I had forgotten to pack my bikini, we decided to go for a walk along the sea front.

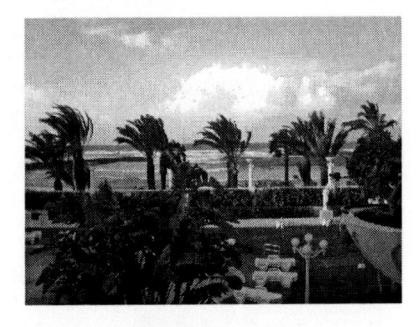

Monday 16

We played at the Amarilla Golf Club, which is situated on the coast and, therefore, affected by the winds coming off the Atlantic Ocean. Today was no exception but I resisted the urge to hit the ball hard into the wind. An eagle three on a par five was the highlight of my round and I am beginning to feel a little more confident with my body to the extent at one point I was told off for jogging on a fairway!

By coincidence Kate and Roger were holidaying near Golf del Sur so in the evening we drove over to see them and went to a local restaurant for dinner.

Tuesday 17

A non-golf day and not renowned as great sightseers – we once toured Washington DC in a day – we drove the mountain route across to Buenavista del Norte on the north-west side of the island to check out a new golf course designed by my hero, Seve Ballesteros. It was my turn to drive and the winding road really put my arm to the test. For most of the journey we were stuck behind two lorries. When, eventually, it was possible to overtake them, I pushed the pedal to the metal only for John to say that the road I had just driven past was the turn we wanted. And men go on about women navigating! Which reminds me – if 90% of all road accidents happen within 10 miles of our home.... why don't we all move 11 miles away?

Neighbours: Steph learns her cancer is in remission.

Wednesday 18

Back to Las Americas again and an easy approach shot to the tenth green with a pitching wedge was painful to say the least. I am not exactly sure what happened but my right elbow and lower arm were not happy with me. I managed to play another four holes before being very sensible and giving in to the increasing discomfort and pain.

Thursday 19
My first period in nearly two months started this morning so I am still unsure what my body is doing as regards the menopause.

Due to a severe thunderstorm last night the course at Adeje was closed. Perhaps it was a blessing in disguise because it meant I could give my aching arm a rest. On the other hand the pouring rain was not conducive to sunbathing and we had spent one day sightseeing. Not wanting to stay indoors we headed north up the motorway as far as Santa Cruz de Tenerife and then picked up the winding coastal road to Igueste and El Bailadero. Although it was my day for driving I magnanimously handed the keys to John. I don't think the gesture fooled him for a single moment.

Friday 20
We drove to Golf del Sur to play a round with Kate and Roger. Everything was ticking along nicely until we reached the thirteenth hole. Instead of playing the easier tee shot down the left-hand side of the fairway, I went for the big carry over the ravine. As I made a solid contact with the ball I felt something go in my lower arm and dropped the club in agony. The thirteenth had proved to be unlucky for me – as I couldn't even hold a club in my hand I had to stop playing. The annoying part was my ball had cleared the ravine and I had a good chance of making par on a difficult uphill hole. Knowing I like a challenge on a golf course, Kate had thought about advising me to play the safe shot but decided I would be sensible enough to think it through for myself and so had said nothing.

Saturday 21
Our last day and we met Kate and Roger at Buenavista for our final round of golf. No buggies were allowed because of two days of heavy rain so we hired trolleys and walked the undulating course. The scenery from the holes near the coastal footpath was fantastic with huge waves crashing onto the

rocks. I played all eighteen holes simply because it was Seve's course and I had taken some painkillers. I guess there was also an element of frustration that my body had let me down again and I had something to prove to myself.

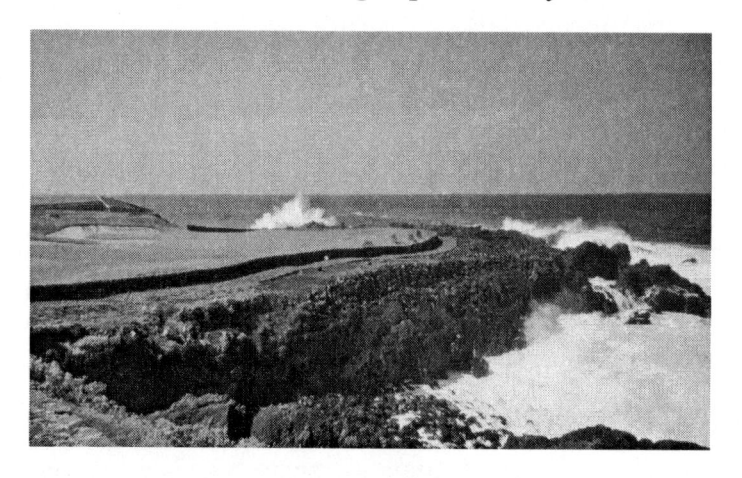

We made it safely to the airport just before the heavens opened and sat in the departure lounge watching the torrential rain. Upon arrival at London Gatwick Airport at midnight, we had to wait twenty minutes in the near zero temperature for the bus to take us to the long stay car park. The sunshine of Tenerife was already a fading memory.

Sunday 22
After just three days and my period has finished. I have decided not to bother about it anymore and let my body do its own thing. There seems little point in wasting energy trying to figure out what is going on!

After a few hours of sleep and breakfast at my parents, we arrived home in time to watch the live football match. It was something of a pacemaker job as Spurs drew four all with struggling Leicester City. For the neutrals I am sure it was quite an entertaining match.

I rang Kate in the evening to arrange some ultrasound treatment on my aching arm.

Monday 23
The diagnosis was a ruptured muscle therefore no golf for a month. Thank goodness I did the damage on holiday and not before it. The ultrasound probe was rather painful as it moved across my arm.

Tuesday 24
More ultrasound treatment today and some exercises to do – Kate is all heart. Afterwards I popped into school for the first time since the radiotherapy treatment started.

Wednesday 25
Kate told me that she had spoken to the orthopaedic surgeon who treated my ankle injury. Apparently the damage I have done has actually saved me an operation on my arm! If I hadn't ruptured the muscle myself it would have to have been cut under anaesthetic to sort out the problem with my elbow. For once I knew what I was doing (not!).

Thursday 26
The Coffee Club, including Point Five, went to Cardiff to visit our former school chaplain who is now training to be a priest. After lunch we walked to Llandaff Cathedral and as we came out it started snowing rather heavily. Back at her college, we sat drinking tea and watched some students build a snowman. I rang John to find out what the weather was like nearer home. Only the baby had a change of clothes with her and I was concerned I didn't have any tablets with me. Around four o'clock the snow stopped falling and we waited to see whether it would freeze or thaw. By six o'clock we decided it was safe enough for me to drive everybody home.

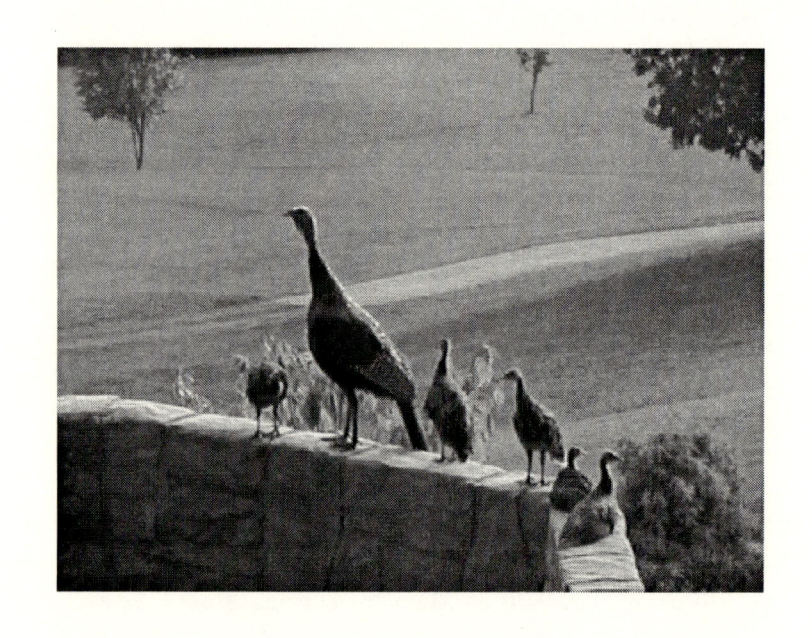

"As we live, so we learn."

March

Monday 1
Very small white patches of skin have appeared on my breast. I pulled at a stitch that has been poking through the edge of the areola ever since the metal clips were removed and felt something tug inside me. Somewhat alarmed I decided to leave the little black thread alone.

In the two months before the operation I lost well over a stone and felt good about my body size and shape for the first time in a few years. I have started to put weight on which must be the side effects of the Tamoxifen. People have expressed surprise when I moan about my weight but, because I have small bones, I appear lighter than I really am. It is the old saying of not judging a book by its cover. I have always been very active and eaten sensibly but a couple of years ago I "filled out" a bit around the waist. I do not want to reach my previous "undesirable" weight again but stopping the Tamoxifen is not a viable option.

Tuesday 2
As I still cannot swing a golf club properly (which is very frustrating) I went for a five-mile cycle ride. My general level of fitness appears to be improving and I have been able to move up a couple of gears on the bike.

Wednesday 3
With various staff absent from school I was asked to help with the Head of English interviews. After four months of not

really having to use my brain it was good to return to thinking mode and mix with staff and students again.

Thursday 4
I drove over to Sue's for morning coffee and a cuddle with Point Five.

Sunday 7
We invited the Outlaws and John's sister and husband round for Sunday lunch. It was the first roast lunch I had cooked for a while and another tick to add to my checklist.

Monday 8
Today is John's birthday and I spent more than usual on his presents; after the diagnosis this was a day I thought I might never see. It is much easier to say this now but, if anything had happened to me, I would have wanted him to start a new life with someone else. One thing cancer has shown me is that life is for living.

I walked into town and back, a distance of four miles, and arrived home in time to catch the health hour on the Jeremy Vine programme on Radio 2. This week's topic was dealing with five different types of cancer. When they reached breast cancer the GP stressed the importance of the five-point self-awareness code (looking in the mirror) rather than self-examination:

- knowing what is normal for you
- knowing what changes to look and also feel for
- looking and feeling
- not delaying in reporting any changes to your GP
- attending breast screening if aged 50 or over

I must admit that, before my cancer, I was unaware of this code and only found my lump through examining myself. She said that the changes that are new or different could include:

- a change in breast size
- a nipple has become inverted or changed its position or shape
- a rash on or around the nipple
- discharge from one or both nipples
- puckering or dimpling of the skin
- a swelling under the armpit or around the collarbone (where the lymph nodes are)
- a lump or thickening in the breast that feels different from the rest of the breast tissue
- constant pain in one part of the breast or in the armpit.

Tuesday 9
I decided on some retail therapy in Street (which sounds a bit hypocritical given my comment last November) as an alternative to watching the rain from indoors.
　　　Sarah rang in the evening to tell me that her second son had passed his scholarship entrance examination and would be joining his elder brother at the grammar school. I was nearly in tears on the phone.

Wednesday 10
An item on the BBC News website:

Breast cancer patients who switch from Tamoxifen to another type of drug halfway through treatment reduce the risk of the disease returning by a third.

A major worldwide trial, co-ordinated by Cancer Research UK, found that women who started taking the drug Exemestane after taking Tamoxifen for around two-and-a-half years were less likely to see the disease recur.

The researchers compared 4700 post-menopausal women – half taking Tamoxifen for five years, which is the common treatment following breast cancer surgery, and the others who switched to Exemestane after two to three years.

As well as finding a 32% reduction in the risk of the disease recurring, the researchers found a 56% reduced chance of breast cancer appearing in the other breast among those taking Exemestane.

Exemestane is a type of drug called an aromatase inhibitor which stops the natural production of oestrogen - the hormone which is responsible for the growth and recurrence of many breast cancers.

Thursday 11
Since Monday's health hour, I have looked at myself in the mirror each morning. In contrast to the left breast, the areola on the right one is now much paler in colour and still concave. Above the breast scar there is a definite rectangle of dark skin, almost like a suntan, which is the result of the booster treatment.

Saturday 13
A long-awaited chance to catch up with some friends from school, I cooked a meal in the evening for ten people.

Sunday 14
The nerves in my right arm were jangling for much of the day. I suppose I did a quite a bit of lifting yesterday and various parts of my body still need time to heal.

Tuesday 16
This morning I was in school to interview the Year 10 students who had applied for the six vacant positions on the Student Leadership Team. At the end of the process I received a message to report to the Head's office before disappearing off site. When I arrived Simon was in there and I was told he needed to speak to me. As he was on the phone I waited outside wondering what on earth he wanted to say. After ten minutes he came out and said we needed to talk in private so we went along the corridor to the interview room. He advised

me to sit down and, metaphorically, my stomach hit the floor. As the third most senior member of staff, protocol required that I should be informed of something before other staff. The colleague in whom I had confided last October and had worked with for nearly twenty-five years, had been reported as missing yesterday, an unidentified body had been found and dental records were being checked. My mind appeared to process the information in just a couple of seconds and, knowing the circumstances when dental records are checked, I could not contain the tears welling up inside. I was conscious of the traumatised nerves in my arm sending out distress signals and that Simon was kneeling on the floor in front of me as though ready to catch me should I fall forward from the edge of the chair with the shock.

Simon rang John on his mobile to ask him to collect me from school and, as I had just been told some devastating news, did not think I should drive my car yet. John arrived within half an hour and Simon explained to him what had happened. We drove home in silence, both of us hoping that the body would not be identified as that of our friend. That sounds dreadfully selfish because, if it wasn't him, someone somewhere was destined to receive terrible news. Later in the afternoon we went for a long walk by the river before retrieving my car.

Wednesday 17
Sleep last night was impossible. Along with many staff I was in school by eight o'clock for a special prayer meeting. Everyone was in a daze but trying to be strong for each other. Remember, no news is good news.

At the end of the prayers one of the science technicians approached me to say that Liz (who lives near her) had slipped a disc, was confined to bed and could I possibly pop over to see her. She gave me the keys so I could let myself in. As my mum once slipped a disc I knew exactly what Liz was going through so off I went on my "mission of mercy".

We spent the day supporting each other and played a few games of Scrabble in an attempt to take our minds off events. The phone call we were dreading came late in the afternoon and we both dissolved. How and why had this tragedy happened?

Thursday 18
I went over to Liz's so that her husband could go to work as normal. Still reeling from the shock we began to reminisce. The phone rang a few times as the office staff kept us up-to-date with information.

Maybe it was coincidence, maybe it was a reaction to the events of the last few days, but my period started today. Perhaps the hormones are settling down and I am returning to my normal cycle.

Friday 19
Although I would not wish a slipped disc (or anything else for that matter) on anyone, I am glad Liz is at home because we have always been able to cry in each other's company and not feel embarrassed.

Sunday 21
About a month ago, in a moment of madness, I agreed to participate with John in a fund raising cycle ride in aid of the local hospital's leukaemic group and other Rotary charities. As the details and sponsor forms arrived yesterday we thought it might be a good idea to drive the cycle route and see exactly what he had "volunteered" us for. We rationalised that the weather was pretty foul so golf was not on the agenda and jobs around the house could wait a couple of hours.

Now, the theory was sound but the practise left much to be desired. The map on the reverse side of the information letter was only a sketch map so we weren't really sure if we were following the correct route or not. However, one thing is very apparent – the event in June requires some serious training if we are to successfully negotiate parts of the Quantock Hills.

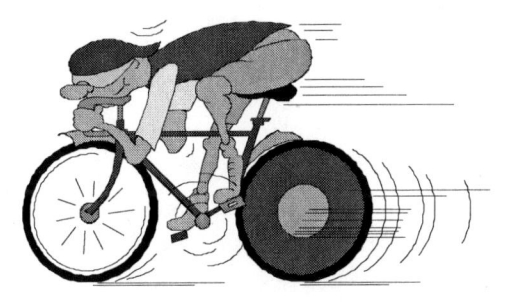

Monday 22
Liz was making some progress and wanted to go downstairs for a change of scenery and lunch, which was fine, provided she promised not to overdo it. The worst part for me was when she decided it was time to return to bed. I said I would keep two steps behind her in case she slipped. "Given **your** current physical state, plus the fact I'm nearly twice your size, that's not very comforting" was the somewhat sarcastic reply. You try to show respect to your elders and help them and that's the thanks you get!

Tuesday 23
My period finished – six days this time, twice as long as the last one.

Wednesday 24
I took a quiz book with me over to Liz's. Two of the tiebreak challenges we tried were naming the fifty states of America and listing all the properties on a Monopoly board.

Friday 26
REST IN PEACE. Today I attended the funeral and am incapable of writing anything even remotely coherent.

Saturday 27
One of the most important days in the year regarding the golf club – The Captains' Drive-In – and I had to withdraw. Apart

from the muscle problem with my arm, I was emotionally drained and the traumatised nerves had been tingling virtually non-stop for over twenty-four hours.

Monday 29
Hormones! Don't talk to me about hormones. Logic tells me that I have made a mountain out of a molehill. That stupid little black stitch poking through my skin has been driving me mad to the extent I have to give it another gentle "persuasive" tug. One second it was inside me, the next it was in my hand with nothing untoward attached. I thought about framing the half-inch piece of thread as a memento and then changed my mind. Is that female prerogative or hormones again? Careful!

Tuesday 30
This evening we went to the Rotary Speaking Competition and dinner – a much-needed, light-hearted distraction from the events of the last two weeks.

Wednesday 31
Mum and Dad's fifty-third Wedding Anniversary. I wonder how many more anniversaries John and I will be able to celebrate.

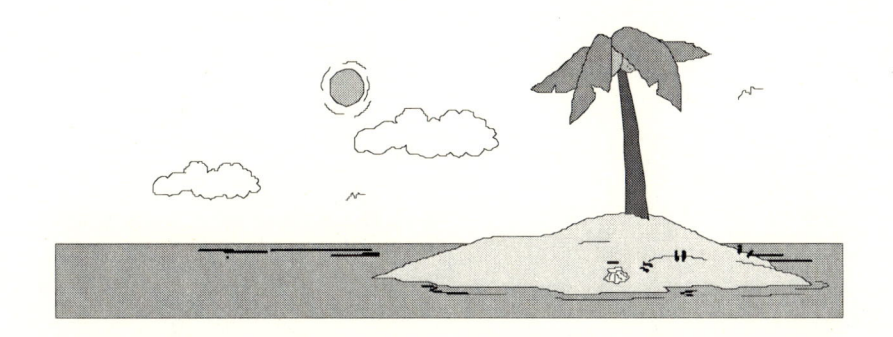

"There are no short cuts to any place worth going."

April – June

April

Conspiracy!
On 20 January I wrote that I did not know how much the cancer had affected John's life but at the beginning of April I found out. He came home one Friday night and said he had a confession to make and hoped I would understand. Some opening line! Recognising my impatience to return to school, he had contacted the other two musketeers to talk about his concerns about both my physical and emotional well-being. Now, we all know about doctor and vicar confidentiality so I have no idea what was discussed. However, John did ask me to consider everything carefully and seek medical advice.

Telling my parents
The Wednesday before Easter I drove the 300 mile round trip to Surrey to collect Mum and Dad. During their week's visit I planned to tell them about the cancer. The next day they wanted to go shopping in Street and, on the way, Dad started talking about my retirement! What prompted this goodness only knows but my immediate reaction was they had worked out I had been keeping something from them.

Twice on the Sunday I thought it was the right moment to reveal my secret and twice I bottled out. Monday afternoon and there was no turning back; I made a pot of tea (standard British drink for all occasions) and, as John took the tray of mugs, I dashed to the bathroom – just the usual problem with my parasympathetic nervous system. On the other hand I think I should definitely take the credit for discovering the cure for constipation! The moment I had been deliberately avoiding for nearly six months and suddenly I felt like a naughty child. With heart in a very dry mouth, I sat beside Mum on the settee and said I needed to tell them something. John was sitting opposite me and nodded encouragingly. I started by saying I had had an operation last November to remove a lump, had tablets to take for five years and had undergone five weeks of radiotherapy at the start of the year. The lump had been detected early, surgery was almost immediate and the removed lymph nodes were clear so the cancer had been confined to one area. I had been into school a few times, done some paperwork at home and we had gone to Tenerife as planned. Dad looked across at John who reassured them that I was telling the truth and was fine.

Mum's first question was had Sarah known about the cancer and I replied yes but she had been sworn to secrecy and they were not to attach any blame to her. Because of your ill health at the time, I took the decision not to say anything and, if it made them feel better, even John had been kept in the dark initially. What's more, if I had to do it all over again, I would take exactly the same course of action. Dad wanted to know about the next phase like how often I would be seeing the consultants for check-ups. Mum's next statement was it would be better for me to take them home on Wednesday as arranged, stay the night and then drive back here Thursday morning. Why? I did the round trip last week when you were blissfully unaware of the situation. Besides, I have an early appointment booked for Thursday.

The next morning, with Mum conveniently having a bath and out of earshot, Dad and I had a chat. He agreed that last November would not have been good timing to tell them my news and I had made the right decision.

Check-up number 1 – the Oncologist
Thursday 22 April and I had my first check-up with the

consultant oncologist. My appointment was scheduled for quarter past six so I spent much of the day expending energy fighting various emotions. I know I should practise what I preach but it is easier said than done. The oncologist examined me and was pleased with what he saw and felt. I cannot say the same was true for me when he touched a rather tender spot and I nearly hit the ceiling. The good news was I did not require any further radiotherapy; just keep taking the tablets.

Sport
Signed off work for the term, I was free to play more golf than usual. I was also asked to organise social fun competitions for Thursday evenings throughout the summer. The middle of April saw my first competitive round of golf since last October. We played in a mixed greensomes competition together and managed to win the trophy. Judging by peoples' reactions when the announcement was made, it was a popular win. It was very emotional as someone commented it was a fairytale ending and the Captain remarked the one person he would have wanted to win was yours truly. Anyway, once I stopped shaking and found my voice, it gave me the opportunity in my acceptance speech to thank people for their support during the last five months.

A chronic ankle injury back in March 1997 left me unable to run for over four years and curtailed my racket sports. The morning of Friday 30 April and I played my first game of tennis since July 1996. Although some of my movement was restricted, the ankle withstood the test of two sets of singles (I had been expecting a doubles match!). During one rally I instinctively stretched for a shot and felt one of the cancer scars pull. However, I survived without any damage and at the end of the match felt pleased that my general level of fitness was improving. Just as well really as I had already promised to have a round of golf with Nicky who had a day off work. Due to heavy rain we only managed ten holes but I felt I could have gone on to complete the round.

Later on in the afternoon I watched the Year 10 boys win the Area Football Cup Final. All in all it was a busy day as I squeezed in the weekly Sainsbury's shopping between the tennis and the golf. Not one to put my feet up before the cancer struck, I may be in danger of overdoing things but there is an inner force driving me to live life to the full. There is no doubt in my mind that I have been given a second chance and I intend to make the most of it.

Survivor

Since my enforced lay-off, I have been emailing two ex-students who were in my first year group. Now in their thirties and both happily married with children of their own, one lives in America and the other just a couple of miles away from us. They were the best of friends at school and have kept in contact with each other and now me. The funny part is that neither of them calls me by my first name even though they left school seventeen years ago and I have told them not to be so formal. Their argument is that it doesn't seem appropriate – even though our relationship has changed, I was and always will be their Head of Year and it is a mark of respect to refer to me as Mrs G. Kids are great and never cease to amaze me! Anyway, "The Local Looney Tune" emailed to say she was again taking part in a fun run for cancer and would I mind if she wore a T-shirt with "I know a survivor" on it. No problems and we agreed to sponsor each other.

May

Check-up number 2 – the Surgeon

Poking and prodding of the various tender spots from the surgeon, much clenching of fists and sharp intakes of air from the patient. In response to my question, he told me the tumour had probably been growing for about a year before I found the cyst, which just goes to show that nobody really knows what is happening inside our bodies especially if we are not experiencing any pain. So that he would have up-to-date x-rays of my breasts he was scheduling a mammogram for me in October prior to the next appointment with him in November. Joy of joys, I can hardly wait for the "M" word and being reunited with the gown!

Training
I have been cycling regularly in preparation for the fund raising ride. One hot Saturday afternoon we went for a ride along the towpath by the river. Because it was flat we cycled about twenty miles and ended up with hundreds of stowaways on our shirts. I have no idea how many actually survived the "flight" but we made a mental note to take bug spray with us next time.

The last Sunday of the month and the weekend before the real event, we thought it prudent to cycle **the route**. After the flatness by the river, the "mountains" known as the Quantock Hills were an experience and just as popular for hitchhiking insects. Perhaps wearing white was not one of my better ideas.

The body not so beautiful
Within the space of five days I played in the Husbands and Wives golf competition and we came second; I played at a course in Devon with three men and they made me drive off their tees; I was involved in the process of appointing our new club professional by being a pupil and having a lesson with each of the four candidates in two hours. By the end of the fifth day, the nerves in my arm appeared to be roasting nicely on gas mark 5!

As for the hormones, what can I say? Attitude – are you telling me I have attitude? Mood swings – you had better believe it! Negative thoughts yes, especially when I am on my own; positive thoughts about myself, not as often as I should. I have experienced hot flushes but, fortunately, not too often;

in the main they have tended to occur when I am uptight about something. Perhaps, in some respects, the Tamoxifen is making the menopause easier for me if, indeed, I am going through it. However, I do **not** like the side effect of putting weight on! Two months in between periods has been great; not knowing when the next one is coming not quite so great. Unfortunately, I have been passing blood elsewhere once or twice a week most weeks and still have not plucked up the courage to consult he whom I know I should consult.

The pinkness of the scars is fading and my right nipple has almost disappeared into the areola; my breast is still tender in places. The booster rectangle has faded slightly but, like the scars, is very obvious to the eye. The cancer has taken away a part of my sexuality as well as my self-esteem; my libido is non-existent. There has been no pressure from John but I feel he should trade me in for a newer, better model. Trouble is I don't think I would warrant any trade-in value.

Music
When I'm at home on my own or driving the car, I like to have noise in the background and am either tuned in to Radio 2 or playing CDs. I decided to make my own compilation CD to listen to whenever I felt I needed the security of being in the comfort zone rather than the twilight zone. Throughout my life certain music has been very poignant so I spent (or was it wasted?) most of a day just listening to loads of CDs before putting these tracks together:

Something In The Air	Thunderclap Newman
The Power Of Love	Frankie Goes To Hollywood
Someone Saved My Life Tonight	Elton John
Here With Me	Dido
Angels	Robbie Williams
Nights In White Satin	The Moody Blues
Total Eclipse Of The Heart	Bonnie Tyler
Everybody Hurts	The Coors

Proud	Heather Small
Just For You	Lionel Richie
Because The Night	Patti Smith Group
Marooned	Pink Floyd
Victoria's Secret	Instrumental from Due South
Lavender	Marillion
Everybody's Got To Learn Sometime	The Korgis
Fields Of Gold	Eva Cassidy

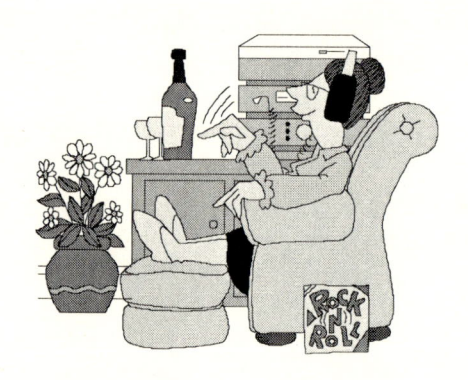

June

News item

Women with breast cancer could benefit from a new technique that reduces some of the side effects from surgery. Currently, when a doctor thinks the cancer could spread, glands under the arm are removed as well as the tumour. But research by scientists at the University of Wales in Cardiff suggests it is unnecessary in two thirds of cases and they have developed a new, less drastic, treatment. The procedure could be widely available in 18 months. Removing the lymph nodes from under the arm is a painful procedure that can result in loss of movement. The research by scientists at the University of Wales College of Medicine found that by removing just one gland from under the arm, specialists can now tell whether the cancer has spread. Using a small dose of radioactivity, doctors are able to locate the main gland – called the sentinel node – that drains directly from the tumour.

Doctors are being trained in the new technique and it is hoped it could be available within two years. Professor Robert Mansel, professor of surgery at the University of Wales College of Medicine, said: "The standard practice at the moment for managing the lymph glands under the arm is that we have to take them all out. The reason for that is we need to know whether the cancer has spread to them. The new technique allows us just to take the most important node - the sentinel node. This means the woman who doesn't have any spread only has a very small operation."

The sponsored cycle ride
Between us we had collected over £400 in sponsorship money. As John decided we would cycle to the start and home afterwards we covered nearly twenty miles. Mind you, he was lucky not to be knocked off his bike by an idiotic Sunday driver who didn't see him on a roundabout BEFORE we reached the start! I was relieved to finish with my body intact.

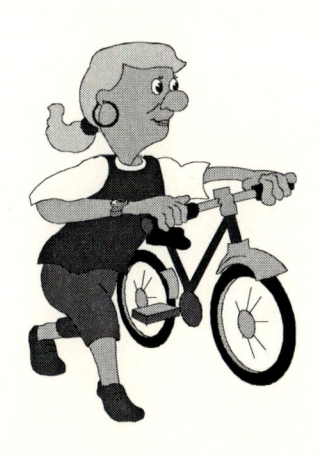

Euro 2004
I entered a fantasy team and hoped it would be more successful than my previous team! England did not start well as they lost to France 2–1 and the jokes came thick and fast.

Why do the English make better lovers than the French?
Because the English are the only ones who can stay on top for 90 minutes and still come second!

Why have all the England footballers been banned from owning dogs?
Because they can't hold a lead!

However, the England team did redeem itself by beating the Swiss 3–0 and Croatia 4–2 and progressed through to the quarter-finals only to face the host nation, Portugal. With the score tied at two all after extra time, the game went to penalties. The records will show England lost 5–6 in the shoot-out. As for my fantasy team – nothing much to report!

Scare number 1
Lymphoedema is a swelling caused by a build-up of lymph fluid in the surface tissues of the body. Surgery or radiotherapy to the lymph nodes in the armpit causes damage to the lymph system, hence the build-up of the fluid. This lymph fluid is important because it contains white blood cells (lymphocytes) that help the body fight infections. The lymph nodes also help fight infection by filtering out cancer cells that have spread from the breast tumour. Some cancer cells will be destroyed but others may escape. Therefore some or all of the lymph nodes are removed during breast surgery to check whether any cancer is present.

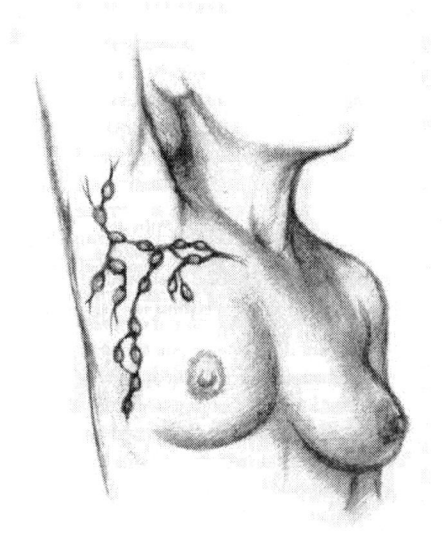

Lymph nodes

Towards the end of June I became concerned about a "lump" on the breast and slight swelling in the right arm so I made an appointment to see my doctor. He examined me and said he thought it was probably scar tissue that had hardened but recommended seeing the breast care sister as a precaution.

I rang the hospital and was offered an appointment for three days later. Arriving at the building where the breast care unit is housed, the nerves were working overtime and, without thinking, I managed to take a wrong turn down a corridor. Realising that I was walking downhill when I should have been going uphill, I retraced my steps and eventually found the right door. I reported to the receptionist who asked if I was there for a screening. No thank you, been there, done that and don't want to go through the triple assessment so soon after the experience of the first one. I'm only here to see the breast care sister.

Apart from examining me, the sister took time to explain about the mechanics and effects of the operation, radiotherapy and tablets. Because I had lobular cancer as opposed to ductal cancer, the tumour was easier to remove but the downside was lobular cancer diffuses more so I had undergone a lymph node sampling. In each armpit there are about 20 – 30 lymph nodes that drain fluid from the breast, the surgeon had removed fifteen of mine and they could not be replaced. Quickly doing the maths I calculated that I had between 25% and 50% of the "plumbing" remaining. She reassured me that the "lump" I could feel was fibrosis and was caused by a build-up of scar tissue – the radiotherapy had hardened the breast tissue – and the swelling was not lymphoedema. I talked to her about my erratic periods and hot flushes and she agreed the Tamoxifen was probably bringing on the menopause. The sister then advised me to examine myself only once a month and, as the operation was just seven months ago, to put the brakes on a bit! Although not worried by what she had seen and felt, she said she would contact the surgeon to arrange a consultation for me just to make sure everything is normal.

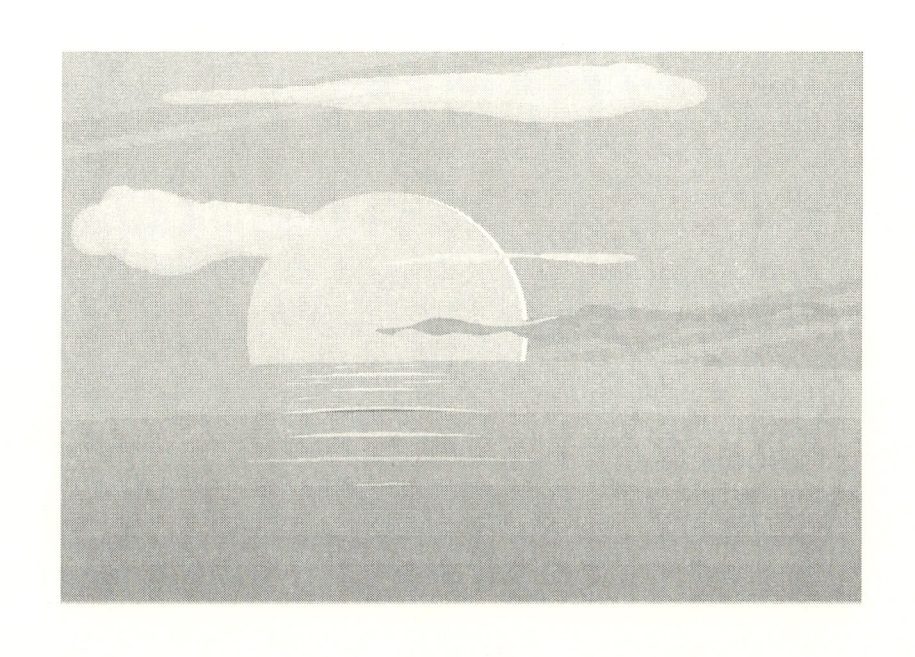

"A smile will gain you ten more years of life."

July – September

July

Godsons number 2 and 3
As well as being an aunt (not that they are allowed to call me that as it sounds really old) I have the privilege of being godmother to my sister's two sons, Tim and Russ. Not being at school this term meant I was free to drive up to Surrey and attend Russ's school play and prize-giving ceremony. Midway through the month Tim came to stay with us for four days to gather data for his GCSE geography coursework and almost ate us out of house and home.

Another book
After twenty years of service to the school, Liz had finally decided to retire at the end of the summer term. A staff social was organised to celebrate her outstanding contribution and I thought it would be a good idea to spring a surprise on her. Aided and abetted by her husband and a few friends, I wrote a "This Is Your Life" book for her complete with incriminating photos!

Check-up number 3 – the Surgeon
The consultant could not feel anything untoward, told me the hardness was due to agitating scar tissue and asked if I had been doing more than usual. Um, can I phone a friend? He also said that the operation was only seven months ago and I had the impression he thinks I am expecting too much of

myself too soon in the recovery stakes. Although there is much to heal, which will require time and a degree of patience, I do not need to stop exercising but be sensible, rest appropriately and take painkillers if necessary. He did say that I had done the right thing seeing my GP, the sister and himself.

Anniversary
Monday 26 July – our twenty-fourth wedding anniversary and I am not the same woman I was in 1980. How could I be? People experience many changes throughout their life but cancer was not a change originally on my agenda. However, it has forced me to take a step back and think carefully about my future and also what is important for John.

August

Golfing holiday in the USA
Much happened during the course of this year's holiday. First of all, everyone and everything arrived at Atlanta Airport, Georgia. Then, courtesy of the internal flight, only John, our suitcase and myself arrived at Myrtle Beach Airport, South Carolina. For the first time in twenty years of golfing holidays, we had been separated from the golf bags. The lost luggage desk attendant at the airport was not at all concerned and said it was a common occurrence for baggage to be sent on the next plane! Eventually our clubs were delivered to us five hours later at half past midnight. Have a nice night, y'all!

Friday 13 August and the weather in the afternoon was not too brilliant so we went shopping to check out the prices on golf merchandise. As we walked around one superstore we heard a sales assistant say that a hurricane was on the way. Yeah, right – 1987, Michael Fish and all that! However, once back at the apartment and the evening television programmes were interrupted by a piercing signal and an instruction to tune into the local station for important information. A mandatory evacuation was in force for people situated east of US 17 but we were staying on the west side and decided to remain where we were.

Saturday 14 August and we watched Hurricane Charley from our condo – an amazing experience. The sheer power of the elements was awesome; telegraph poles were blown over as though they were mere matchsticks. At one point I watched a deer and its fawn come out of the woods and stroll down the adjacent fairway before disappearing into the trees again. The electricity was out for four hours but the cable TV went off for nearly a day so we were unable to watch the USPGA. We went shopping instead for golf shoes, balls, gloves and a pack of cards each, as you do! Consequently the luggage home was rather heavy.

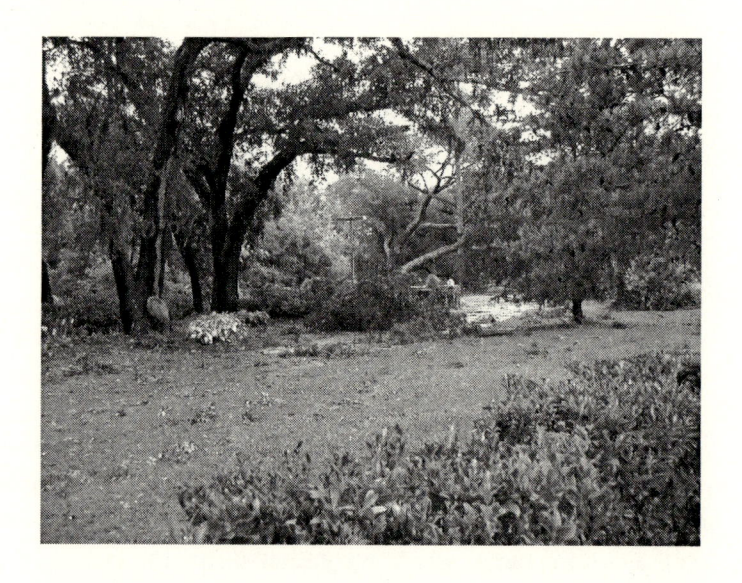

Friday 27 August and we were in Atlanta to watch the Atlanta Braves play the San Francisco Giants. The baseball game was good and we bumped into a friend and his wife from Springdale (the course where we stay in the Great Smoky Mountains) there. Given the size of both Turner Field Stadium and the crowd we thought that was pretty remarkable.

Sunday 29 August and I had a hole-in-one on the 144 yard par 3 second hole at the Lakemont Course, Stone Mountain Park near Atlanta. The professional is sending me a certificate as a memento. As I have now aced a hole in North Carolina (Blue Ridge Country Club, 26 August 2000) and Georgia, I have decided to go for acing a hole in each of the remaining forty-eight states – Alaska could be interesting. Based on my current performance of an ace once every four years, I should complete the task in 2196 at the ripe old age of 241. Forget the Oscar, I could become an entry in the Guinness Book Of Records!

Our flight back home was delayed for two hours due to a thunderstorm so we didn't arrive at London Gatwick Airport until half past eight on Bank Holiday Monday morning. I have never suffered the effects of jetlag travelling to or from the United States, which was fortunate as the next day was the thirty-six holes Ladies' Championship postponed from July. Although the temperature was twenty degrees cooler than on holiday, I adapted quickly and managed to retain the nett salver trophy I won last year. However, three and a half weeks of golf almost every day and my arm had built up some excess fluid. Perhaps, in hindsight, I overdid things just a tad!

September

The 35th Ryder Cup
Kate and Roger joined us for three days of nail-biting tension. Never mind the players feeling the tension – we must have played every shot as well but it was worth it. The European team was victorious on American soil and there was the bonus of Monty sinking the winning putt. Yes! It doesn't get much better than that.

My birthday
Sunday 26 September. Next year is the *0 all being well!

News

Chemoprevention (prevention using a drug) studies are currently being undertaken to look at whether drugs can be used to prevent breast cancer in women who are at high risk of developing breast cancer.

The largest of these studies, IBIS I, (International Breast Cancer Intervention Study I) looked at whether the hormone treatment Tamoxifen can prevent breast cancer in women at higher-than-average risk of the disease. Preliminary results have shown that the incidence of the disease was reduced by one third in women taking the drug. However there were several side effects associated with Tamoxifen, including increased risk of endometrial cancer and hot flushes. Therefore, Tamoxifen is not normally prescribed for breast cancer prevention.

IBIS II is a new trial to compare Tamoxifen with a new hormone drug called Arimidex. It is for women who have been treated for early stage breast cancer, or who have a higher-than-average risk of developing the disease. Arimidex works in a similar way to Tamoxifen, but is believed to have fewer side effects.

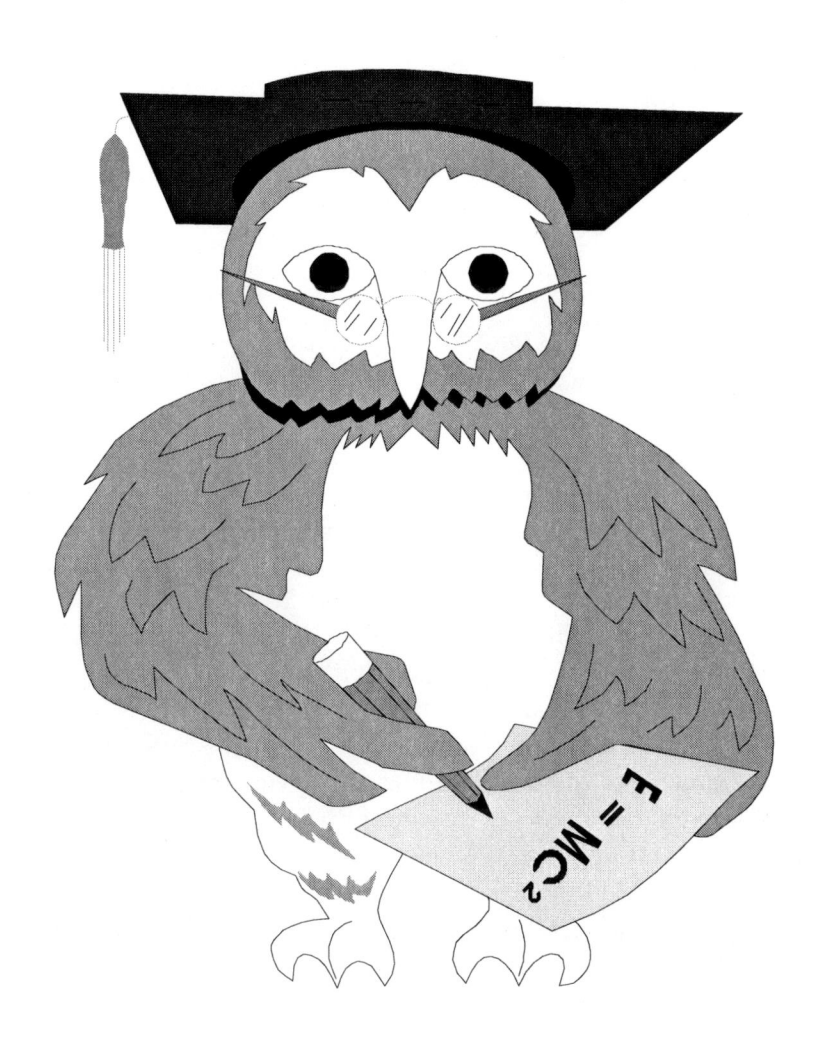

"Today is the tomorrow you worried about yesterday."

October – December

October

The next phase of my life
Friday 1 October and today is the beginning of the next phase of my life. But, and it is a huge but, the beginning of what? For various reasons I officially resigned from school yesterday and I now have this enormous void to fill. I also have to somehow deal with all the questions and emotions spinning round my head. Did I let my body down or did it let me down? Either way I feel angry with myself because I am not superhuman any more. I feel incredibly vulnerable and fragile to the extent I cannot let anyone else become really close to me, not even John at the moment. Why did this have to happen to me? I always tried to give 110%. What did I do wrong? Having resigned I am also left with this deep sense of guilt and abject failure at letting so many people down – the kids, their parents, staff, family and friends. Who am I? When and how will I ever get my identity back? It is difficult to describe the feeling of much pain and sense of loss deep within; I have some secrets which must remain secret. So many questions and no easy answers; I reread the cards whilst listening to the Comfort CD and, afterwards, restored the mask.

Return of the mammogram
Wednesday 27 October: after many months of withdrawal symptoms, I was reunited with my favourite item of clothing –

the fashionable surgical gown. The radiographer asked me a few questions and explained what she was going to do; I resisted the urge to say I have been here before so please just get on with it. I asked her to do the left breast first as I knew what was coming. She said that, in my position, she would have chosen the other side first in order to get it over and done with. The right breast was painful to say the least (as I knew it would be) and made my eyes water especially when I had to stretch my arm out and almost cuddle the machine. However, the radiographer was very considerate and ran down the room to press the button and then ran back to release me. She told me to put the gown on while she went to look at the x-rays and warned me not to leap to conclusions if she returned and asked to do another set of mammograms but the machine could be a little temperamental at times. As I sat clutching the gown around me, my mind drifted back in time to the day of the triple assessment. I wondered how life had treated the three knitters I saw at the hospital just over a year ago. After ten minutes or so, the radiographer returned to say I could go and get dressed. I now have to wait a week for the results and have a real fear of what I may be told.

Janet
Thursday 28 October and we attended Janet's funeral; the church was full of people whose lives she had touched. As the pallbearers rested the coffin on the trestles I could not hold back the tears. Someone said that God only takes the best. Sadly, He decided the time was right to do just that.

November

Check-up number 4 – the Surgeon
Thursday 4 November: I have been well and truly prodded today as the surgeon found all the painful spots. He managed to find one bit I didn't know existed but do now! I have had some pain in the breast and it is where most of the tissue was

removed. It could take at least another year to settle down but I am not to stop any arm movements. The golf and tennis will continue to be painful at times but I can live with that. At least I have an idea of what is going on inside my body and these twinges are nothing untoward.

Last week's mammograms showed that the right breast was normal for what I have had done but the cysts have returned to the left side. Although he is not concerned at this stage he wants to monitor the situation and see me in May, have another mammogram in October before a check-up in November. I was really hoping to have a year's exemption from hospital visits but it is not to be.

Fantasy football
Monday 29 November and I received an email informing me of my Fantasy Football Manager of the Month Award for November. I have won a pair of football boots and a football so look out Tim and Russ! Apart from the success in the league, I had five wins out of five in the UEFA Cup competition and my squad has a bye into the next round. Not bad for a girlie and a definite improvement on my previous fantasy teams!

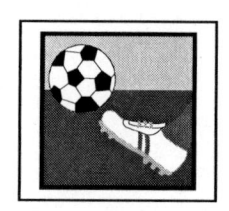

December

Scare number 2
Wednesday 1 December and it is eleven months since we went to see Return Of The King and I first passed blood. It has been an on-going problem but today I passed considerably more blood than usual. With John away in Newcastle on business, Kate had invited me over for a meal before taking

part in a quiz evening. Scared by what had happened, I rang her to ask if I could go round earlier than planned. Upon arrival, she immediately asked what was wrong, made me a cup of tea and, as we sat in the kitchen talking, I had a partial sense of déjà vu.

Thursday 2 December: I consulted the person I should have consulted months ago. He rang through to his secretary and asked if she would make an appointment for me with the appropriate consultant. Oh boy, here we go again!

Monday 6 December: at the surgery for blood tests and I remembered being told to avoid having my blood pressure or blood samples taken from the right arm as an infection or injury to the arm on the treated side could slightly increase the risk of developing lymphoedema. The practice nurse was excellent as I never felt the "slight scratch" and easily managed to fill three phials with blood. Obviously my left arm is not as reluctant as my right arm when it comes to giving away the red liquid. Before leaving, she wished me good luck and sincerely hoped I had nothing to worry about.

Wednesday 8 December: in hospital for the bowel cancer test. First of all I was given a phosphate enema and suffered a bad reaction. I nearly passed out in the toilet and had three nurses around me at one point. Needless to say I am one of a small minority of people who have problems with these particular enemas. Once I was feeling better the consultant arrived, apologised they had made me feel unwell and then performed a flexible sigmoidoscopy (the nurse gave me the leaflet to read afterwards!). This was definitely not an experience I ever want to repeat because it was particularly painful, especially when the tube appeared to reach my throat! Good news though – no bowel cancer, just haemorrhoids. I was offered the opportunity to have the band ligation done there and then or to return next week. Next week? No way, José, while you are here please feel free to do what you have to do.

The nurse who was with me most of the time knew about the breast cancer and I think she guessed my fears about having bowel cancer. We had a chat about various things and I mentioned the book I was attempting to write about my experiences. Today's events would obviously be mentioned. She told me about a personal tragedy she had experienced in her life and said: "I really believe He only puts on the shoulders of those who can cope and give something back to others. Keep on writing."

Christmas 2004
Christmas Day and we had "Old People" for lunch – well, it made a change from the usual turkey! My parents were staying for five days and John's mother and stepfather joined us. One of my presents from John was an MP3 player so I can now record up to eight hours of music. Should keep me entertained on future long-haul flights. Next year sees our Silver Wedding Anniversary and we are planning to make a special trip to Canada. After all, there will be much to celebrate.

DENTAL SURGERY

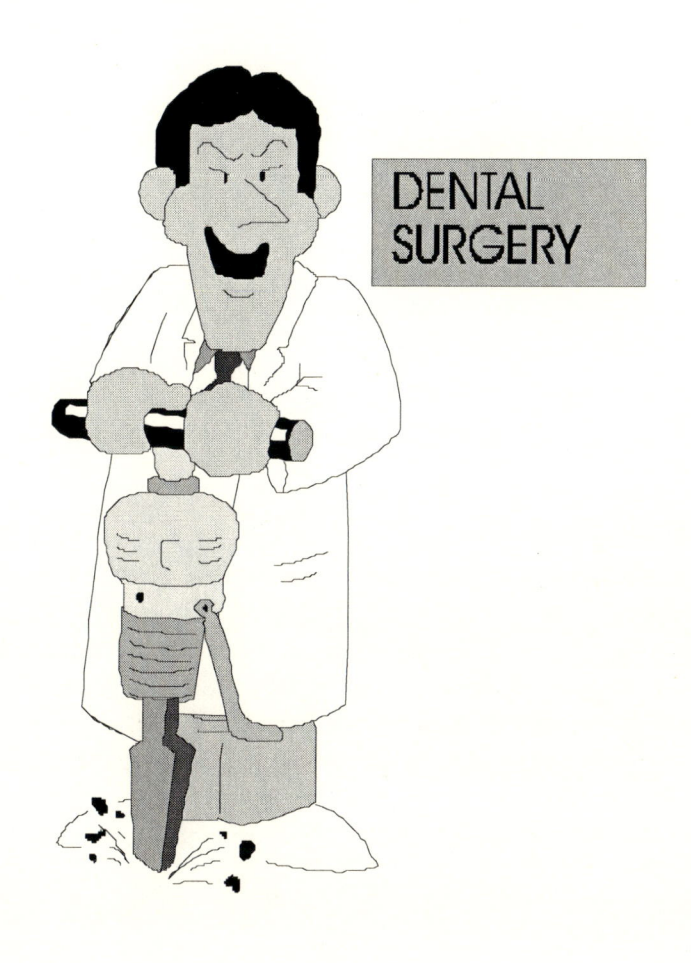

"May your troubles be as few and as far apart as my Grandmother's teeth."

Life Afterwards

So, there you have it – over a year and a half of my life that started with stress related symptoms and then hit me with the dreaded "C" word – cancer.

Life is full of experiences, some good, some not so good, but it is how you react and what you learn from them that is important and, hopefully, makes you a better person. It is amazing what you find out about yourself, your family and friends especially in the face of adversity. We all possess an inner strength to help us through difficulties but should never underestimate the power of support from those around us. Nobody can predict the future so we need to make the most of the here and now and take nothing and no one for granted. I have definitely overdone things at times – played tennis when the arm was aching, cycled up hills when perhaps I could have walked part of the way, played golf virtually every day for three weeks but I suppose I had a point or ten to prove to myself and everyone else.

I have learnt much about life and myself in general. I promised my sister that I would be around for many years to come and I fully intend to honour that promise. Everybody told me I had the right attitude to the cancer and was always positive about recovering completely. However, I would be deceiving the entire universe if I said I hadn't gone through some very dark thoughts and days. Because I never felt ill at any stage, I am not sure I ever fully accepted that I had the disease. Perhaps it was an unconscious act of bravado, perhaps I was in denial – maybe I will never know. I do know that I desperately wanted to protect those around me, especially John and my parents, and often had a mask in place when dealing with people. Sometimes I knew instinctively that I needed space to myself and then felt pangs of guilt afterwards for shutting people out. I was overwhelmed by the support I received from family, friends, colleagues, students past and present and their parents; in particular I must single out the Three Musketeers. Perhaps the most emotional statement came from a golfing friend who said I had been to hell and back but everyone was glad to have back the person they knew and loved. It was both powerful and very humbling.

Someone I knew was having radiotherapy at the same time as me but, for her, it was her second round of treatment – her cancer had returned to a different part of her body. She also had to undergo chemotherapy. I was always honest with her when she asked me questions about how she looked etc. because I wanted people to be honest with me. Honesty was the best policy for me because I could then deal with situations in my own way.

The frightening statistics are that one person in three will develop cancer; one woman in nine will develop breast cancer. Some medical staff said I was too young to have breast cancer but everyone has a cancer cell lurking somewhere – it is a question of what triggers it off. Stress is a highly subjective state of mind that is difficult to quantify and there is no clear evidence as yet that stress increases the risk of developing cancer. Living my life the way I did for the three or four years prior to my diagnosis was not living at all and would probably defy the Trade Descriptions Act! In hindsight, my natural instinct to care for people meant I was working hard to be all things to all people and completely ignoring my own needs. As Simon once said to me martyrs don't win prizes here on earth. I realise he was pointing out in his usual forthright manner that I had lost all common sense in the pursuit of attempting to help everyone except number one. I now try to avoid stressful situations as much as possible as I firmly believe that was my trigger. However, that is easier said than done especially when the Inland Revenue starts communicating with you! But that is another story for another time (maybe). I do appear to have developed a warning system that kicks in if I allow matters to get on top of me. Either the traumatised nerves in my right arm start sending out distress signals or I feel very hot. It would be foolish of me to ignore these signs in the future. I still have no idea whether I am menopausal or not but I manage to live with the Tamoxifen by counting down the remaining months to "demob Tamoxifenication". Although I am physically fit and well, my sexuality and self-esteem continue to be a problem and I cannot see the light at the end of these particular tunnels yet.

The one certain thing in life is death and I consider I have been given a second chance to live. My priorities have changed as I feel I have cheated a death sentence and become a member of an exclusive (but, sadly, ever growing) club. That may sound very dramatic but if, dear reader, you have also been through the mill I think you will understand what I mean.

People have asked me if I am in remission. None of the medical staff has actually mentioned that word to me so I don't really know the answer but, on the positive side, I was lucky my cancer had not spread to the lymph nodes. The risk of developing the disease again is highest in the first five years – hence taking Tamoxifen for that length of time to reduce the chances of the cancer cells returning. Advances in medical science and technology are being made – nowadays the majority of women with breast cancer are successfully treated. More women are living longer with breast cancer due to earlier detection, more effective treatment and better care.

We have to believe that cancer can and will be beaten. Paraphrasing The X-Files duo, Mulder and Scully – the cure **is** out there.

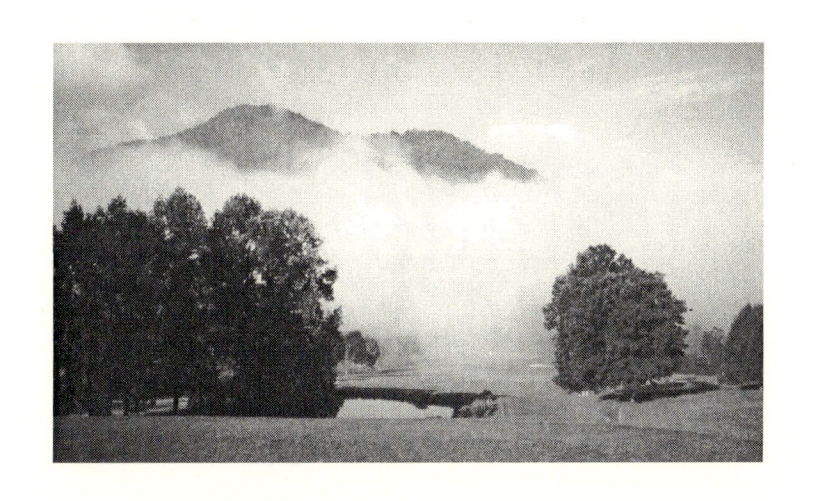

It is not about what if,

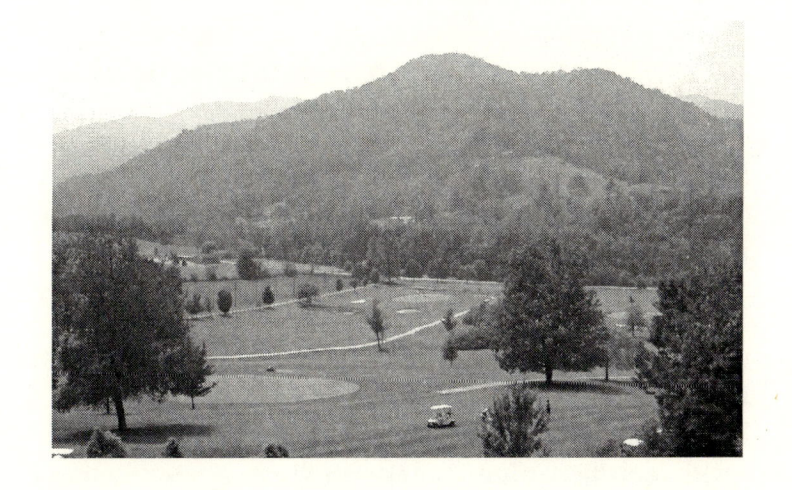

it is about what is.

John's Memories

I can vividly remember sitting with my mother, in our front room, being told by a consultant that my father had inoperable cancer. I was twenty-one and a university student at the time. My memories of sitting beside my father's bed as he died three months later are just as vivid twenty-seven years after his passing. On both occasions I can recall a feeling of numbing despair that I never envisaged having to cope with in my life again.

However, when I came home from a week's business trip to Ireland and found that Mamma had discovered a lump in her breast, there was nothing in my past that could have prepared me for the emotions I was unexpectedly subjected to. Less than a month earlier I had been to my 49 year-old cousin Liz's funeral. Liz's illness had begun with breast cancer.

Mere words cannot begin to describe the emotions I found myself suddenly experiencing. Underlying all these emotions was a fear I had never known before. The sudden possibility that your soul mate, best friend and partner, in every respect, might not be around is something you do not consider when you are still in your forties.

Over the next twelve days I went through a roller coaster of emotions, which included despair and anger, but the fear never diminished. Surprisingly, the turning point came with the consultant's words to Mamma "I'm sorry to tell you that you have breast cancer...". Deep down I think I always knew what the diagnosis would be. The confirmation meant that I was able to focus on fact instead of possibilities and in a position where I could concentrate more on listening to the proposed plans for her treatment. I would be lying if I didn't admit to the sharp pain in the pit of my stomach.

Finally knowing meant I could begin to absorb the remainder of the consultation. I picked on the positive aspects of his words, in particular that he believed that the cancer had been caught early and that there was a good chance of a full recovery.

This was by no means the end of the trauma but, from then on, I was more able to focus on planning the future and ensuring on "being there" and doing what I could to get us through it. By taking things one step at a time Mamma overcame a number of personal hurdles and came out the other side in a manner that made me really proud.

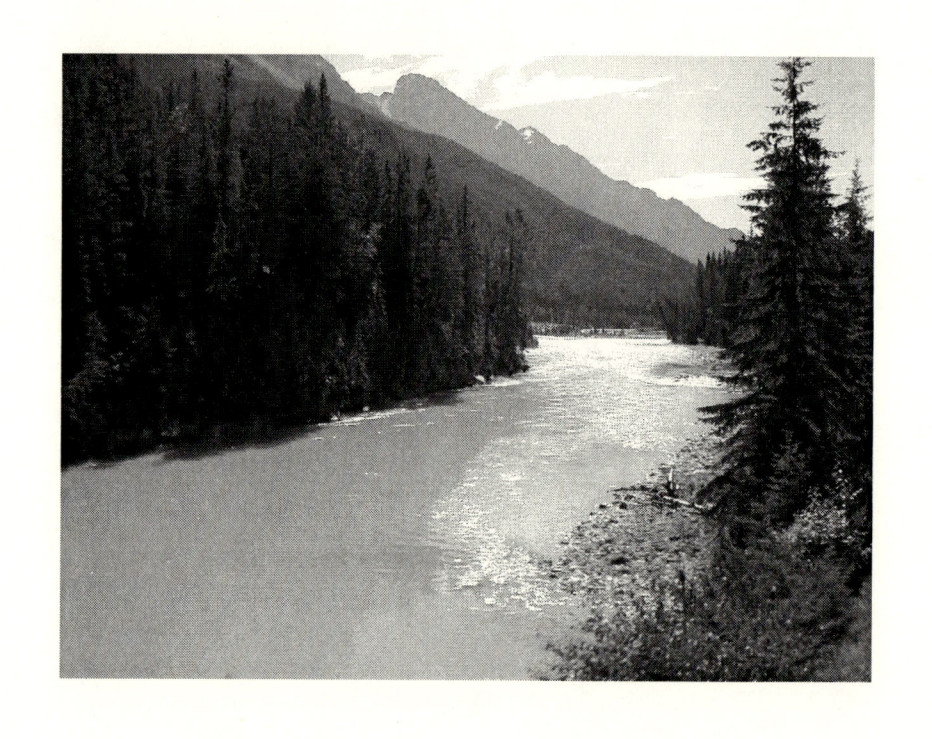

"Yesterday is history.
Tomorrow is a mystery.
Today is a gift.
That's why it's called
the present."

Epilogue

July 2005

Godsons number 2 and 3
Tim enjoyed his visit last summer so much that he asked if he could stay with us again and chill-out after his GCSE examinations and subsequent work experience week. Due to the forthcoming anniversary celebrations he stayed for ten days instead of the original five and I visited Sainsbury's several times to keep up with his incredible appetite. At least an inch taller than last year and not an ounce of fat anywhere, I felt as though I was feeding the proverbial bottomless pit. We took him to our golf club for a round of golf and he caddied for me in a competition and for John in the Pro-Am so he earned his keep – well, some of it!

As a sports shop in town had a closing down sale, Tim and I went shopping for new trainers and football boots. What an experience – my sister had forgotten to warn me how particular he is regarding clothes and footwear. As the car park ticket neared its expiry, we hadn't bought a single thing so I dashed off to put in more money. Eventually he found a pair of boots he liked and also bought goalkeeping gloves, shin pads and a golf glove, bargains all, so I guess it was worth spending two hours in just the **one** shop!

Halfway through Tim's visit, my parents arrived for a week's holiday and Russ for a four-day sleepover, the idea being they would be extra hands to help with the party preparations. Russ was impressed with his brother's sports purchases so I offered to take him out for some retail therapy. Oh boy! Fussier than Tim, nothing was suitable and, suffice to say, I have put it down to one of life's experiences all aunts should undertake just the once. However, unable to accept defeat and being a glutton for punishment, our second attempt the following day was more productive and expensive; in fact, within twenty seconds of entering the shop, he had spotted a shirt and asked if he could try it on as he wasn't sure of his size. The next fifty minutes was happily spent with me bringing him various shirts and shorts to try on. We eventually left with two shirts, a pair of shorts, shin pads and a pair of football boots! The boys definitely take after their father when it comes to buying clothes. I had an email from Sarah thanking me for teaching her sons how to shop and sparing her hours of frustration!

Silver Wedding Celebration
Saturday 23 July and we had all the immediate families (bar one nephew who was in France on holiday), our Best Man, his wife and two of their three children here to help us celebrate our Silver Wedding. We also renewed our wedding vows and Simon led a short service in our back garden. Before the service I visited the bathroom three times – my usual problem of the nervous system taking over – and even had to ask Simon to delay the start for five minutes while I disappeared. Sarah read I Corinthians 13 (a reading of much personal significance since leaving my secondary school ** years ago) and John's sister a poem called "Silver Anniversary". Very appropriately, Simon's address centred round a golf ball – it has no beginning or end, no edges bar an inside and an outside, it is dimpled and designed to travel. Much like marriage – it is designed to have no beginning and no end on earth, it is to have no edges bar the depth of things kept inside it and those that are outside for all to witness, experience and see. Marriage is intended to travel; it is a journey that when two become one they travel together. A journey that two commit to not knowing where it will take them or where they will find

themselves on the way; for better for worse, for richer for poorer, in sickness and in health as the vows say.

At the end of the service, Simon removed his dog collar and joked that I hadn't wanted the barbecue lit earlier in case people thought they were attending a cremation! The heat from the coals was so intense that James, who was helping John with the cooking, managed to "brand" his stomach with the metal buckle from his trousers belt. In between feeding the assembled masses and ensuring glasses were topped up, I did manage to eat something myself which is more than I achieved at our wedding reception! The wedding photographs were on display and most remarks related to the fact that nobody had seen me wear a dress since that day.

Silver Wedding Anniversary
Tuesday 26 July, our anniversary and, before taking part in the thirty-six holes Ladies' Championship, we opened cards and presents from family and friends. John caddied for me and, as people assembled in the clubhouse prior to the presentation of trophies to the prize-winners, he served everybody with a glass of champagne. Apparently he had arranged this with the Bar Manager a couple of weeks ago as an anniversary surprise for me.

August

Saturday 6
Canada here we come!

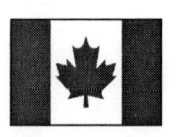

We flew from London Heathrow Airport to Calgary, a distance of 4364 miles according to our information pack. (As we usually fly from Gatwick Airport, this was only the third time we had flown from Heathrow – the first was on our wedding day to our honeymoon destination of Yugoslavia and was John's first ever flight.) Having adjusted the watches to

Mountain Standard Time and collected the hire car we successfully navigated our way round the outskirts of Calgary and on to Canada 1. As we passed the site of the 1988 Winter Olympics, we imagined Eddie "the Eagle" Edwards standing at the top of the 70 and 90-metre ski jumps. The flatness of the edge of the Prairies eventually gave way to our first sight of the majestic Rockies and we also spotted a moose standing in a creek. We found our hotel in Canmore and, as we stepped out of the car, the smell of the fir trees was powerful and the view of the mountains breath-taking. Having literally dumped the luggage in our room we drove into the town in search of a supermarket, as you do. My first and lasting impression of Canmore will always be the 4-way stops at the umpteen crossroads. Canadian drivers are so polite – everyone sits there and waits for everybody else to make the first move. Thank you kindly!

Sunday 7
Our first round of golf on Canadian soil was at Banff Springs. Amazingly the girl at the bag drop came from a town twenty miles from where we live. The world really is shrinking. Apart from the spectacular mountain scenery, we saw white-water rafters (including a dog wearing a bright red lifejacket) and an osprey catching a fish in the Bow River that flowed beside the course. We also had to fight off chipmunks that persisted in leaping onto the golf buggy in search of food. One chipmunk was so frustrated with his/her lack of success that a "calling card" was left!

Monday 8
Silver Tip (the local name for a grizzly bear) Golf Course and the mountains appeared to be even bigger and better. The course has gone straight to the top of our all-time top ten list although we were disappointed not to see a bear.

Tuesday 9
We drove to Kananaskis to play the Mount Kidd course and

had our first sight of coyotes in the wild as two of them strolled nonchalantly across the course in front of us. Like Banff Springs, the combination of mountains, trees, river and wildlife was simply awesome.

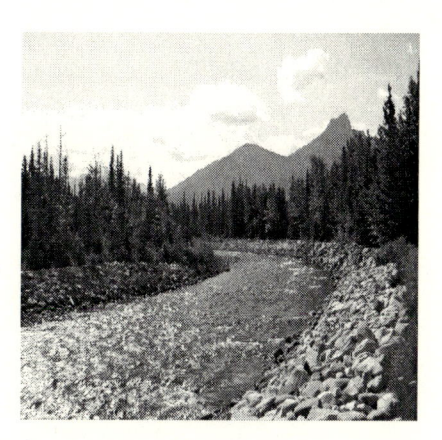

Wednesday 10
After yesterday's sunshine, shorts and 80^0F, we were reduced to wearing the waterproofs for the entire round in an attempt to keep warm as the temperature had dropped thirty degrees. Even the elks seemed to be taking shelter in the woods from the bracing wind.

Thursday 11
The Rocky Mountaineer is billed as "the most spectacular train trip in the world" and who would argue against that statement? The first day and the train took us the 309 miles from Banff to Kamloops (derived from the Shuswap Indian word "T'Kemlups" meaning the meeting of the waters) the junction of the North and South Thompson Rivers. In-between the many awesome sights of the mountains we saw a helicopter airlifting a bear to a new location; the Wapta Lake (wapta is the Stoney Indian word for river) which is the source of the Kicking Horse River; the Spiral Tunnels – an incredible feat of engineering whereby the railway doubles back upon itself twice in order to cut down the gradient of the railway from 4.5% to 2.2%; the mouth of the Adams River which is the site of the world's largest sockeye salmon run; and finally the Hoodoos, the name given to the unique rock and clay formations formed after the last ice age.

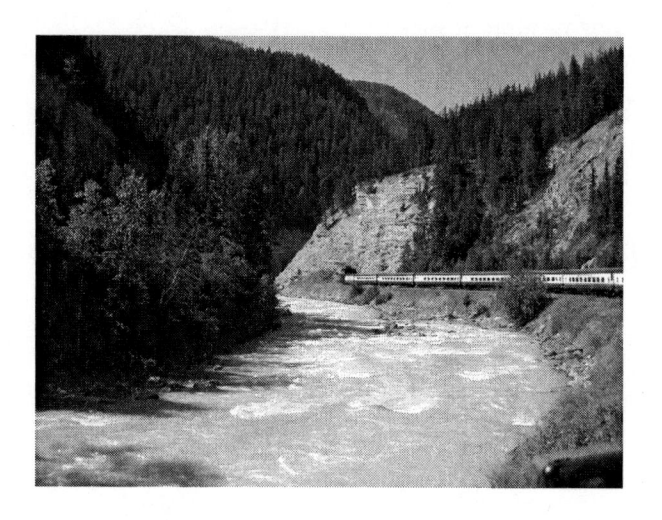

Friday 12

Day 2 on the Rocky Mountaineer and we travelled 276 miles from Kamloops to Vancouver and into another time zone, the Pacific Standard Time. As we left Kamloops Kim (one of our coach attendants) gave us a list of wildlife to look out for during the journey. Like millions of parents or teachers trying to keep children entertained on long trips, I am convinced this was just a clever ploy! We did see ospreys (fish eagles) and bald eagles but the bears, moose, mountain goats and wolves were conspicuous by their absence. However, to see the natural beauty of formations like the Rainbow Canyon, where the minerals in the rocks reflect a rainbow of colours and give the canyon a painted appearance, made up for the lack of animals, as did Lytton where the Fraser and Thompson Rivers meet – we could see clearly the distinction between the muddy Fraser River and the clear water of the Thompson Rivers; and Hell's Gate, the narrowest part of the Fraser River where 200 million gallons of water pass through a 110 feet wide gorge every minute.

The last two days have exceeded all our expectations, especially the superb cuisine, and we would love to do the reverse trip sometime. Actually, tomorrow would have suited me but we had to drive from Vancouver to Whistler Mountain, site of the alpine and Nordic venues for the 2010 Olympic and Paralympic Winter Games, for the next stage of our holiday.

Sunday 14
We played golf with a Japanese couple, which was great fun as they couldn't speak English and my Japanese is limited to counting from one to ten. On the fourth hole a golf ball hit me, full force, on the top of my left thigh. As I sank to my knees in pain, Mr Japanese raced off in his golf buggy to tell (presumably in sign language) my "attacker" what had happened while John put some ice in a towel. I'm not renowned for putting ice on injuries but today was an exception. Suddenly people were arriving from all parts of the course. The group ahead of us had actually heard the impact of the ball on flesh and had called the pro shop for assistance before coming over to see me; Mr Japanese came back with the couple we had played with yesterday – Mr American was beside himself at the thought he had hit someone he knew. A member of staff then arrived with a bag of ice and to check whether medical personnel were required. I decided it was time to take matters into my own hands, told the others to finish playing the hole, then stood up and started slowly walking around. I played the remaining par threes and fours but sat in the buggy with the ice on my leg on the par fives.

By the middle of the afternoon I had a bruise the size of a saucer and a huge lump at the point of impact. However, the sunshine was beckoning so we decided to take the gondola to the top of Whistler Mountain. I'm very glad we did – the views were stunning.

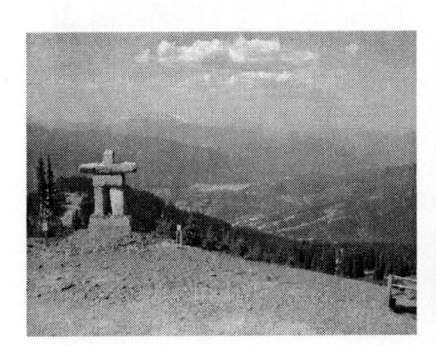

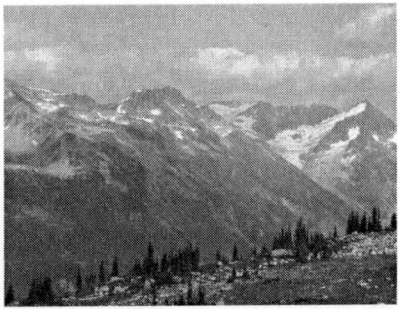

Wednesday 17
After breakfast we took our time driving down the scenic Sea to Sky Highway back to Vancouver, stopping to take photographs along the way. Our hotel room overlooked the harbour so we could watch the numerous seaplanes taking off and landing; we also had an uninterrupted view of Grouse Mountain. We had dinner at a restaurant by the harbour-side and heard the famous Nine O'clock Gun being fired from across the water at Stanley Park. I've decided that Vancouver is a city I could happily live in.

Thursday 18
We hired bikes and spent a relaxing day cycling round Stanley Park and building Inukshuks from stones we found on the beach before boarding the evening Amtrak to Seattle.

Friday 19
America

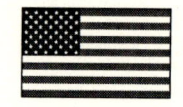

The Space Needle apart we left Seattle wishing we had spent another day in Vancouver.

Saturday 20
We flew over two thousand miles to Atlanta and into our third time zone of the holiday, the Eastern Standard Time. As soon as we stepped out of the terminal, we were hit by the familiar humidity of Georgia and the fresh air of the Canadian mountains was a distant memory. Bring on the air conditioning for the drive to the Great Smoky Mountains of North Carolina. After the magnificent Rockies, I have to say that the Appalachians appeared to be mere hills.

Wednesday 24
11.10 p.m. and we were just about to turn the bedroom light off when we felt the room shudder. At first we thought someone was trying to force open a downstairs door but the

shuddering continued for over twenty seconds; our next thought was perhaps we had experienced an earthquake.

Thursday 25
The local TV news confirmed that a minor earthquake measuring 3.8 on the Richter scale occurred last night and we were about twenty-five miles from the epicentre.
     GCSE results day and a phone call to Tim to learn he had achieved ten passes at the top two grades. I had to swallow several times so that my voice didn't break with emotion.

Sunday 28
During the overnight flight from Atlanta to Gatwick I calculated that we had travelled (via planes, trains, cars, bikes) nearly twelve and a half thousand miles through four time zones, two Canadian provinces and walked and/or driven in three American states. It made a change from counting sheep.

Tuesday 30
I had been asked to give a talk about my radiotherapy experiences and decided to read part of the book to the assembled masses. Although I'd practised reading the selected diary entries aloud, I found my voice breaking with emotion at times. However, I was encouraged by people's positive reactions and comments afterwards – many of them had no idea what treating cancer involves. On a personal level I guess certain aspects of my illness are still very raw and the healing process requires more time. There again, I never was a patient patient!

October

Tempus fugit – mammogram and gown time!
Friday 14: I was sitting in the small reception area awaiting my annual mammogram and experiencing the usual problems

with my nervous system when one of the bar staff from the golf club walked out of Examination Room 1. The nurse who helped me through the bowel cancer test saw me, smiled and said hello before taking Helen to see a consultant. As the radiographer who did my mammogram last year called me in to Room 2, I crossed my fingers that Helen was at the hospital for a check-up and nothing more sinister.

This year's mammogram was no less painful on the right breast than it was twelve months ago. Whilst the radiographer was out of the room checking the quality of the x-rays, my mind began to wander over the events of the last two years and I hoped Helen was not about to embark on the same journey.

November

Check-up number 6 – the Surgeon
Thursday 3: the six months since check-up number five in May have passed in the blink of an eye. I was told that the latest mammograms were clear and then the surgeon asked me some questions about my periods, any reactions to taking the Tamoxifen and family history regarding anyone suffering from osteoporosis. As I haven't had a period since March and not experienced any adverse problems with the tablets, he concluded I was postmenopausal and, therefore, ready to change to a different hormonal therapy. The new medication is called "Arimidex" (I've heard that name before somewhere) so I will have to go surfing again with Jeeves on the Internet.

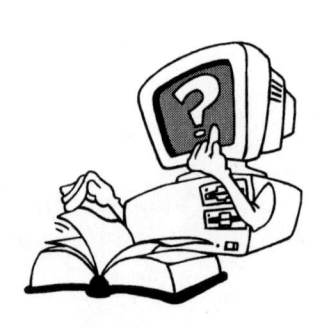

Anastrozole is a type of hormonal therapy used in the treatment of breast cancer in women who have had their menopause. Many breast cancers need supplies of oestrogen in order to grow and in women who have had their menopause, the main source of oestrogen is provided through the conversion of androgens (sex hormones produced by the adrenal glands) into oestrogens. This is carried out by an enzyme called aromatase and the conversion process, known as aromatisation, happens mainly in the fatty tissues of the body. Anastrozole blocks the process of aromatisation and reduces the amount of oestrogen in the body. Therefore, it's goodbye to Tamoxifen and hello to Arimidex for the next three years. Oh, and it's goodbye from me as well. Take care!

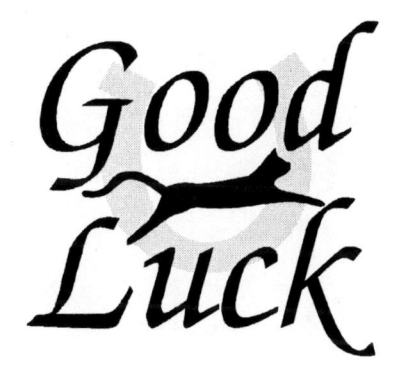

Good Luck

Still wishing you everything you wish yourself.

Mamma Gram
January 2006